I was Poisoned by my body...

The Odyssey of a Doctor Who Reversed Fibromyalgia, Leaky Gut Syndrome and Multiple Chemical Sensitivity —Naturally!

* * *

Gloria Gilbère, N.D., D.A.Hom., Ph.D.
Foreword by Merry Alto, M.D.

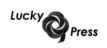

Fourth Printing: February 2004

Lucky Press, LLC
126 S. Maple St.
Lancaster, OH 43130
740-689-2950
www.luckypress.com/poisoned
books@luckypress.com

PRINTED IN THE UNITED STATES OF AMERICA ON ELEMENTAL CHLORINE-FREE PAPER WITH SOY-BASED INKS.

Cover design: Deborah Vicari
Illustrations: Tama Bergstrand, Beata Golau
Interior design: Rosamond Grupp
Editors: Prof. Howard Waterman, Jan Scott, Sonja Beal, Janice Phelps

Publisher's Cataloging-in-Publication
(Provided by Quality Books Inc.)

Gilbère, Gloria. 1947-
   I was poisoned by my body : the odyssey of a
doctor who reversed fibromyalgia, leaky gut
syndrome and multiple chemical sensitivity,
naturally! / Gloria Gilbère. -- 1st ed.
    p. cm.
    Includes index.
    ISBN: 0-9676050-9-1

    1. Gastrointestinal system--Diseases--
Alternative treatment. 2. Naturopathy.
I. Title.

RC827.G55 2001   616.3
            QBI00-500057

This book is dedicated to:
Muffy and her mother, who made this book possible and
taught me, by example, the true meaning of "unconditional."

You, the reader, for taking this step
in pursuing natural health-care.

Dedicated practitioners of the healing arts and pioneering
physicians who have the unprejudiced and inquiring minds
to search for true causes of disease and drug-free therapies
and, when found, the courage to proclaim and offer them
for the benefit of their patients…even when the healing
modality is contrary to currently accepted traditional
consciousness and practice.

In loving memory of my paternal grandmother...
my first "natural healer"

IMPORTANT AUTHOR UPDATE

With this new printing, it's important to keep in mind that the recommendations and therapies mentioned within are to be used as guidelines — every case is unique. Since my recovery from the disorders discussed, many new products and healing modalities have come to light, many of which were not included in this publication, yet are now, however, recommended in my consulting practice.

Five years after *I was POISONED by my body...*

Many clients and readers have asked if I have fully recovered. When you consider my current lifestyle consisting of the following, YOU DECIDE:

- I maintain a private clinical practice and consult both at my health center and via telephone with clients, physicians and researchers around the world
- I've written five more books since the first printing of this book — *Invisible Illnesses; Nature's Prescription Milk; Living with MARS: Multiple Allergic Response Syndrome; Cooking and Living without Inflammation;* and, still to be released, *Prescribed Addiction: Not What the Doctor Ordered.*
- I have a weekly web-based radio show on www.healthylife.net.
- I write monthly for seven major natural health magazines.
- I am president of the local chapter of the American Ballroom Dancers Association.
- I make an average of 14 trips per year to lecture, teach and attend conferences.
- I completely remodeled a home to my "non-toxic" specifications with no health challenges.
- I sit on the advisory board for the Fibromyalgia Coalition International and Library of Health.
- I consult and formulate products for neutraceutical companies.

Do I live a "normal" life without limitations? That depends on your perspective of what normal includes. I still do not consume foods in the nightshade family because of their propensity to induce inflammation; I keep myself away from toxic situations (fragrances, petro-chemicals, pesticides, mold etc.); I wear a mask while flying (a healthy proactive approach); I eat in restaurants with attention to ingredient details; I maintain a detoxification protocol; and I enjoy life, giving thanks every day that I was able to reverse the life-threatening course on which I was thrust — subsequently becoming the health architect for those who also choose to build their health, *Naturally.*

Contents

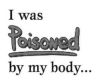
Foreword: Merry Alto, M.D.

It is humbling to have a patient with devastating illness and, despite all the years of education and training, be helpless in finding the cause and treatment for the illness.

It was almost one year ago when the author of this book—a highly educated and experienced alternative medicine professional—came to me with near anaphylactic-like allergic reactions to nearly all foods, hair loss, insomnia, myalgias, arthralgias, and profound fatigue. No test I did elucidated the cause. No treatment I gave helped, and in fact only compounded the problem.

Dr. Gilbère researched her problem from the alternative medicine viewpoint and began treatment. Within a few weeks, the hair loss stopped and within a few months she looked healthier than I had ever seen her. The results were incontrovertible! I was astounded!

Fortunately, we do not see each other's educations and treatments at odds with each other, but rather quite complimentary—each contributing something valuable to the care of our patients.

Please read Dr. Gilbère's personal case report. I can verify her remarkable results and encourage both mainstream and alternative medicine professionals to consider the leaky gut syndrome when faced with a baffling complex of patients.

—*Merry Alto, M.D.*

President, Washington State College of Emergency Physicians, American Association of Physician Specialists, Association of Emergency Physicians, American College of Emergency Physicians

Foreword: Lola Righton, D.A.Hom.

What if nearly every morsel of food you put in your mouth, the odor of every passing vehicle on the street, walking down the aisles in the grocery store, the chemical smells of new furnishings and clothing in department stores, outgassing from familiar items in your own home, and using cleaning and personal-care products you've used for years suddenly causes your throat to swell so that you can't swallow and can scarcely breathe, your face to turn beet red, hot and swollen, rashes and welts to erupt over your body? What if this is a daily occurrence? Several times daily? Your entire world has turned against you. You are assaulted by invisible chemicals and their odors on every hand, each triggering a violent response in your body over which you have absolutely no control.

Why is your very existence suddenly threatened by your environment?

Multiple chemical sensitivity is a problem of modern times. It affects all of us, even those who don't manifest the violent responses of the "canaries" in our society. Allergies to foods or chemical substances, both the ones your body is able to respond to and those to which it no longer can—anti-inflammatory drugs; antibiotics and adverse effects of many other pharmaceutical drugs; chemical exposure in the home, on the job, or elsewhere; and ravaged immune systems—each of these or in combination can make you vulnerable to severe nutritional deficiencies, digestive breakdown, and erosion of the protective mucosal coating of the bowels. Trashy particles of fecal matter are absorbed directly into the bloodstream. You have the symptoms of "leaky gut."

Viewed under a microscope, your blood would look like a sewer . . . and it is. No wonder you feel so awful.

Too many of us, when we find ourselves ill, rush to the medical community and lay ourselves at their feet, saying, "Here I am. Heal me." It's just not that simple.

The answers are not solely to be found in the printouts of the laboratory analyses, in the results of tests performed by various expensive pieces of equipment and interpreted by those trained in their small sphere of application. The search for health is complex. Success is not instantaneous and the road is arduous and physically, as well as emotionally, painful. Once lost, health is not easy to recover. It requires personal involvement, research, and perseverance.

It takes courage to pick up the unraveled strands of what is left of your health, discover the tools you need to begin knitting them back together, and then create and evolve your own instruction book. Dr. Gilbère has done this. It wasn't to impress anyone. It was to save a life, her own.

We have been colleagues in the field of alternative medicine for many years and have consulted on the more thorny problems of our clients and shared details of each other's health challenges. After returning from what had promised to be a relaxing vacation, Dr. Gilbère called me in great and increasing pain. We discussed it over the telephone and, at the time, could come to no conclusions regarding the suddenness of its onset or the persistent and debilitating effects on her life and practice. In the following pages, she recounts her increasingly desperate search for relief from the relentless, piercing pain, the consequences of conventional medical treatment, and her struggle to survive.

There is a terrible emotional toll on the sufferers of "leaky gut" and related syndromes. Many of you out there are without support from family and friends who simply do not understand how someone who looks so normal from the outside can be in such misery. Your symptoms are often varied and seem unconnected by any conventional view, but are in fact related by their root causes. It can be very lonely out there wondering if, as you are no doubt sick of hearing, "It's all in your head." Reading this book may be a tremendous relief. You are not alone. You are not a "head" case. Your symptoms are real. There is a way, and here is the guide to assist you. Someone who has been down that road and knows the dark corners personally has compiled her story of research and recovery and how she incorporated it into her busy, pressured life.

To say, "I don't have time for that, I can't afford that," is not much of an excuse when the quality of the rest of your life, not to mention life itself, is at stake.

Dr. Gilbère is an example of someone who lived solely on organic rice products and variations of fresh organic carrot juice supplemented by vitamins, minerals and natural remedies for months at a stretch when her body would tolerate nothing else without violent reaction. Every introduction of new foods was by baby steps: If there's a reaction, stop! Go back! Wait a week or so and try again. Over and over again this was the way she inched back into eating a slightly more varied diet. I'll never forget her excitement over having successfully consumed, with no reaction, an organic yam! Or her first scrambled, organically-raised egg! Everything that crossed her lips had to be organically grown. That meant creative solutions to the lack of local availability. She couldn't go to the corner health-food store in her very small town and find everything she needed. Living this way, having to be so very careful of your food supply, not having the luxury of dining out, brown-bagging your lunch every day, having to take your own food to a friend's dinner party or when you travel, soon becomes commonplace.

Oddly enough, when you are forced to make such radical changes in your eating, you are doing yourself a huge favor. Your overall health is bound to improve just because you are no longer polluting your internal environment with the toxic chemicals that pervade our conventional food supply.

Dr. Gilbère struggled through the food issues, and just when she thought it was safe to face the world again—wham! The fumes of traffic on the roads in town seeping into her car on the highway; the smells emanating from the new computer in her office; outgassing of new carpets and furnishings in her home; the chemical smells at the hairdressers; being exposed to fragrances—all began to close off more and more activities and made her examine, evaluate and modify her surroundings very care-fully. The new computer could only be operated for a few hours and then shut off to reduce the chemi-cals it emitted. Road trips had to be limited or eliminated altogether. Visits to the hairdresser had to be curtailed. Does this sound familiar? Is this what's happening to you?

For my own part, sitting on the sidelines has been very illuminating for me as a health practitio-ner. Tracking Dr. Gilbère's progress through the use of colon hydrotherapy has been an eye-opener for me. I had always been greatly prejudiced against the use of enemas and similar treatments as being more damaging than helpful. Some clients I have known were so habituated to their constant use that they could scarcely have a successful bowel movement without laxatives and enemas. Colonics and colon hydrotherapy were lumped together in my mind and in the same boat as laxatives and enemas. Dr. Gilbère's evolving program of treatment incorporated colon hydrotherapy and colon cleansing by means of special herbal-bulking agents. The obvious observable beneficial changes were at times dramatic, especially following an allergic reaction. After many months of shared information, I have begun carefully recommending this type of program to certain individuals.

The fatigue, pain, hunger, misery, and fears experienced and shared by her have developed a greater empathy and, I hope, sensitivity in me with friends and those who consult with me. Her journey and anguish have already served hundreds, and will, I am sure, serve thousands more. The journey is not over, but it is a lot further down the road than it was. Dr. Gilbère's odyssey can serve as a source of information and encouragement to the many sufferers of "leaky gut" syndrome and the related illnesses.

Have courage for your own future, for your life. Take charge of your own health! Choose to be well. Read this book.

—*Lola V. Righton, D.A.Hom.*
Diplomate, Academy of Homeopathy

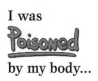
Acknowledgments

My business partner, Sharon Wiseman, for her unending encouragement, support, and tireless hours spent "keeping me keeping on." Without her this book would not be possible. Most importantly was her insistence to turn my medical challenges from "bitter lemons" into "healing lemonade" and make it available to all who want the recipe.

My healing mentor, Lola Righton, who unselfishly gave of her expertise, time, energy, and friendship to open the doors to the world of homeopathy and then guided me, and pushed when necessary, to make sure I walked through.

The following people who shared their professional knowledge, time, and expertise: Anne Plante, Regina Danielsson, Beata Golau, Rhea Maloney, Russ Holt, Riley Livingston, Dr. Merry Alto, Dr. Marshall Arbo, Dr. Christopher Sturbaum, Dr. Marty Becker.

My extended support group, who listened, encouraged, shared, and cared: Lew and Jean Mace, Tiffany Francis, Earl and Helen Heinemann, Louie and Adeline Arroyo, Cristina Mendez, Don and Mildred Campbell.

My organic network for providing me with organic food, and to my delight, introducing me to foods and preparation methods I'd never heard of: Donna Marie McCandless, Joan Myers, Gregg Prummer, Marsha Semar, Bill and Ruth Wagner, Debbie Ackley, and the many clients and friends who shared from their organic gardens and orchards.

My publisher, Lucky Press, for seeing the value of my work and their ongoing support to continue my writing.

Prof. Howard Waterman, who took time from his demanding schedule to edit, encourage, and tutor.

Jan Scott, whose expertise in editing was a Godsend. She endured my naivety of computers, problem-solved, and spent countless hours organizing my writing.

Tama Bergstrand, for her friendship, and commitment to perfection, so evident in her illustrations.

Beata Golau, who through her professional expertise, compassion and sensitivity not only fine-tuned my body, but, with her brilliant illustrations, interpreted my insight and experiences.

Author's Note

I have been in the profession of health-care for more than thirty years and, as a practitioner and facilitator of natural health, have consulted with thousands of clients worldwide, assisting them and their physicians to design a road to health, Naturally. The focus of my work is education and research in non-invasive methods of identifying and correcting health imbalances: physical, psychological and environmental. Being in the profession of natural health, I am proud to set an example of "practicing what I teach." The following is an account of how, after a life-threatening accident, I fell into the same cycle of symptom-care as so many of my clients. I share my in-depth experiences and solutions on the road to quality health, naturally.

An Important Note

This book introduces alternative therapies for leaky gut syndrome and the associated disorders. It is written to help you understand, assess, and decide appropriate treatment for a given disease or condition. The author does not intend to make comparisons between traditional and alternative medicine, other than in the context of personal experiences.

Therapies in this book are based on the training, experience, and research of the author. Because each individual is so unique, the therapies may or may not be appropriate for you. This book is not intended to replace proper medical care. Do not stop taking medications without talking to a physician or health-care professional. If you decide to use any of these approaches, take this book to a physician or health-care practitioner and request the appropriate tests. If a health-care professional will not, or cannot, order the requested tests, seek one who will honor your request. It is your right to obtain a second or third opinion. Take personal responsibility for your health by becoming well-informed regarding available therapies.

Because any therapy can have risks involved, the author and publisher are not responsible for any adverse effects or consequences resulting from the use of any of the suggestions, products, or procedures described in this book.

This book is not intended to diagnose, treat, or cure disease, nor to prescribe, nor be a substitute for, medical care. Rather, it is intended to share experiences and research and to be used as an educational tool.

Introduction

This book is the first of its kind to directly connect the causes of autoimmune disorders, allergies, inflammatory diseases, and multiple chemical sensitivities with colon and digestive disorders. It outlines the gut causes of, and therapies for, chronic illnesses frequently misdiagnosed or un-diagnosed. It offers safe, alternative, natural choices to drug therapy.

We have become a society that expects instant results instead of taking full responsibility for our health. Doctors and health-care professionals are physicians, not magicians. The information provided here *will* assist you in making informed choices because, after all, it's you who must live with the consequences of those choices. If your attitude is "give me a quick solution to get rid of my symptoms," alternative medicine is not for you. If, however, you are "sick and tired of being sick and tired" and willing to work towards health, this book is the road map for your journey. The medical principle, "Do no harm," is honored by many of both the newer and more ancient concepts, that are non-invasive. These alternative therapies have little possibility for harm and can be extremely effective.

The new paradigm in health care involves active consumer involvement and responsibility *in their own* health care. It involves openness on the part of patients and their physicians, both abandoning their narrow, restricted, "quick fix" attitudes and looking deeper for causes. It requires a change of attitude, honoring the ability of patients, as consumers, to think for themselves and know their bodies. It relinquishes the practice of disease-care, with its subsequent symptom-care, to health care.

It involves a shift in belief to accept the concept of wholistic health, the whole person as mind-body-spirit. It embraces wellness as what we eat, how we digest it, how we utilize it, what we believe and think, and how we move our bodies.

My Story:
Surviving on Carrot Juice and Rice
Is NOT Living!

Six years ago I survived a life-threatening fall. As a result, I developed what was medically diagnosed as chronic fatigue and, eventually, fibromyalgia. I struggled for several months with prescription-drug side effects. The medications provided very little relief and served to bring on a new barrage of symptoms.

I eventually regained my quality of life through alternative medicine and wholistic therapies. I was *not* prepared for what followed.

I was overdue for a long weekend respite. A colleague invited me to spend a few days in the desert. It was the middle of winter in northern Idaho, and a visit to the desert was hard to resist. On the second day of my trip, I was sitting in a movie theater when suddenly I experienced inexplicable acute pain in my right shoulder and a radiating pain from the back of the right shoulder blade (thoracic area). My right hand went numb, finger mobility was lost, and the pain was intolerable. Had this been my left side, my gut feeling would have been "cardiac." My tenaciousness helped me physically get through the film; however, my medical mind was preoccupied searching for a probable cause. The pain continued through the evening, varying in intensity. The next day, acute swelling manifested at the bottom of my neck. I looked and felt like the hunchback of Notre Dame. The pain in my right shoulder blade felt like a piercing rib, and I felt as if I were walking around with a bowling ball strapped to my neck. Just holding my head up took enormous effort.

Four days later I flew home, and, for the next four weeks, I consulted with my allopathic medical doctor, chiropractor, and massage therapist, without improvement. Cervical and thoracic X-rays were taken to diagnose any structural injury. No evident cause could be found for this debilitating pain and swelling. After five weeks of escalating pain and impaired function, I reluctantly agreed to prescription drugs for pain management and inflammation. Shortly thereafter, I noticed my throat felt internally swollen, with no external evidence. I could swallow, but it was restricted. I mentioned these symptoms to my physician, who then suspected thyroid malfunction. A thyroid-function test showed normal levels. The swelling didn't escalate, but it was chronic, with few days between that were symptom-free. Then another symptom emerged . . . my hair was falling out in alarming quantities. Previously, I had enough hair for two women and was very proud of it. Having witnessed this toxic drug effect in my clients, the fear of going bald escalated as my medical doctor and I kept digging for an apparent cause. It is now obvious we were looking in the wrong places.

This vicious cycle of pain, swelling, and drug side effects continued for four months. My medical doctors were as puzzled as I was. My next referral was to a neurologist to evaluate for spine involvement. The MRI showed massive swelling in the thoracic region, but no apparent functional cause. My medical diagnosis was "thoracic outlet syndrome." At this point, while still attending to my practice, in acute pain, and with little quality of life, *I again, reluctantly agreed to prescription drug therapy.* I was prescribed a strong non-steroidal anti-inflammatory drug (NSAID). The pain was manageable with the NSAID; however, the following side effects manifested within one week: acute constipation, abdominal cramps, bloating, accelerated fatigue, muscle pain and weakness, heartburn, "thickened throat," and heart palpitations. The symptoms were a daily occurrence. My family, friends, and clients observed the steady decline of my health. I had helped hundreds of clients overcome side effects of prescription drugs, and now I was in the same vicious cycle. Modern "wonder drugs," with their toxic side effects, took another victim, *me.* I had spent most of my professional life searching for quality health care with safe and effective alternatives. Now I was caught up in the same web as my clients before they sought a wholistic approach to their health.

After four weeks of taking the NSAID, I started to experience rashes in reaction to foods I normally consumed. The reactions manifested as profound red, hot, flushing welts in my face and neck. At times my eyes were barely visible through the swollen lids. In addition, the rashes would appear as an apparent cause of having an empty stomach. I knew the hot rashes weren't female mid-life "power surges." Anxiety set in. I had witnessed this reaction in my clients with food allergies, but I didn't have food allergies, at least not before these drug side effects. I believed I had a "cast-iron" stomach. How could I suddenly be reacting to the food I had consumed for years?

Six weeks after starting the NSAID, while eating a sandwich, my throat began to swell. I could hardly swallow. With panic in my voice, I called my medical doctor. It was conclusive I was having anaphylactic

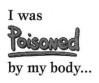
shock and needed immediate medical care. *(I had a flashback of symptoms reported by my clients that had sent them running to the hospital emergency room.)* Subsequently, a prescription was given for an antihistamine drug and an anaphylactic injectable kit with the drug epinephrine (adrenaline), used for bee and insect stings. In retrospect, a drug, not an insect, had stung me. I took the prescribed medication only to have the same effects: repeated throat closures accompanied by progressive intensity and panic.

The next option proposed was a steroidal drug to control the reactions. I opted to forfeit any more drugs, especially steroids. It was now clear how patients get caught in the tangled web of prescription drugs and their side effects.

In addition, a new symptom developed: insomnia. This time, unlike the previous sleepless episodes caused by fibromyalgia, the insomnia was acute. This was chronic fatigue, of the mind and body, at its worst.

I was afraid to eat. The same food causing a reaction one time did not provoke one at another. I would try only vegetables; some triggered a reaction and others didn't. Every time I attempted something new, I'd blame the reaction on that food group. There weren't a lot of foods left to experiment with, and the symptoms made me more and more afraid to try. After extensive research and consultation with professional colleagues, I initiated a diet plan to cleanse and support the body while identifying the offending foods. From past experiences with clients, I suspected leaky gut, but still didn't have confirmation. I resorted to a diet of freshly juiced organic carrots, apples, ginger, and rice. This proved to be the best tolerated and least reactive.

The weight loss started. Within two months I eliminated forty pounds. I could surely use the weight loss, but not this way! As if this wasn't enough, my hair continued falling out in chunks, my previously clear complexion now had acne and rashes, and my nails developed deep ridges. Another manifestation of my malnourishment and liver stress were dark circles under my eyes and a yellow color to my skin and eyes. Traditional liver-function testing results were "within normal ranges." However, alternative testing showed excessive liver stress and inability to neutralize toxins. The chronic fatigue and muscle soreness made me feel as if I was bruised all over.

As the condition progressed, I became more and more isolated from family and friends. I couldn't go anywhere without carrying my organic juices and rice. I had no energy to socialize. It took all my energy to continue my practice, return home at the end of the day to prepare food I could tolerate, and fall into bed, though not to sleep. My nightly companions were pain, tears, and helplessness. Frustration was coupled with flashbacks of all the clients who shared similar stories of symptom-care. This was not living; it was surviving. Most nights I couldn't even muster enough energy for a valued telephone conversation. Some friends and family kept asking, "Aren't you better yet?" So I stopped giving any details when asked, "How are you doing?" No one understood, unless they, too, had experienced an illness that forced a complete lifestyle change.

Some people thought I went too far by refusing to eat anything nonorganic. Those were the people who weren't with me, or someone else, in the midst of a violent reaction to nonorganic foods. No, I

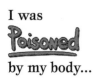
hadn't become a health fanatic. I was struggling for survival. I took pride in maintaining my reputation as a gourmet cook, but didn't cook exclusively organic. My meals were low-fat and balanced, using organic foods from my own gardens and buying locally-grown organic produce and poultry, when available. Now, nonorganic was not an option; it was essential to life. The addition of chemicals in the food, either for growing or preserving, could kill me.

The winter months in northern Idaho were the most challenging and expensive. I couldn't go to my local grocery store and buy organic foods and produce. All produce had to be special ordered at a health-food store forty-five miles away, purchased in the closest metropolitan city 125 miles away, or purchased frozen through a co-op delivery service twice a month.

My primary-care physician did everything possible within the range of traditional medicine. I am fortunate in having a medical doctor who listens to her patients and then goes the extra mile to facilitate solutions. Many times, her solutions include referrals to alternative-medicine practitioners, even though it may go against the traditional consciousness of her peers. Much to her credit, when all she could offer me was more medications for symptom-care and another traditional referral, she said, "I have no answers for you. You know more about this condition than I do."

The next suggested traditional referral was to an allergist to determine which foods and substances I was allergic to. I had been down this road with many clients who had never fully recovered because the root causes were never dealt with. I was in a vicious cycle of *symptom-care, not health-care.* Disease had set in. I was again on a professional quest, this time it was for me. So . . . I set out with the determination of a health detective to find the *gut* of my disease.

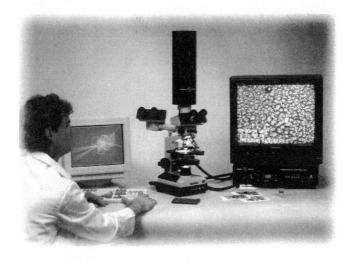

My suspicion of leaky gut syndrome grew, but I needed to see it for myself. I scheduled an innovative blood test called a live cell analysis. I previously had this test performed on a yearly basis as a way of monitoring my health (yearly check-up). It is accomplished through a single living drop of peripheral blood taken by a laboratory technician or practitioner from the fingertip onto a slide. It is then put under a powerful microscope, magnified up to 12,000 times, and transferred to a computer monitor by way of a fibre optics camera for the patient to observe. The patient is intimately involved by being able to see the immediate test results (the true essence of living color), usually explained by the technician and/or practitioner.

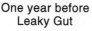
Live Cell of Colon Area

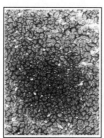

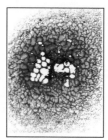

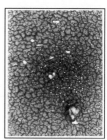

| One year before Leaky Gut | Showing Leaky Gut and inflammation | Ten months after healing from Leaky Gut |

My suspicions were confirmed: leaky gut. The above photos identify the condition in the area of my intestinal tract before developing leaky gut, after developing leaky gut, and the healing that occurred ten months later. This is a case where a picture is truly worth a thousand words, to the patient and to the health-care provider. Unfortunately, traditional medicine in the U.S. does not generally use this testing method, although it is widely used in Europe, Australia, Japan, and Latin America.

Now that I had a definitive diagnosis, I saw that my body was poisoning itself. Armed with this information, I started the journey of my life, to find appropriate natural therapies providing real solutions, not band-aid drugs, to heal and regain health, naturally.

Today, I'm on the road to wellness (with a full head of hair—a little grayer for the wear), along with the many clients who seek my help in their gut-wrenching journey to *add life to their years, not just years to their life.*

1

What is Leaky Gut Syndrome?

Leaky gut syndrome (LGS) is a clinical disorder associated with increased intestinal permeability. Simply put, large spaces develop between the cells of the gut wall. It's like a damaged or destroyed digestive filter that allows bacteria, toxins, and food to leak into the bloodstream.

The official definition is an increase in permeability of the intestinal mucosa to luminal macromolecules, antigens, and toxins associated with inflammatory degenerative and/or atrophic mucosal damage. Essentially, it represents a hyper-permeable intestinal mucosa or lining.

LGS causes inflammation of the intestinal lining and damage or alteration of the microvilli (cellular brush borders lining the intestinal tract). The damaged cells (microvilli) are then unable to produce the necessary enzymes and secretions essential to effective digestion and absorption of nutrients.

This increasingly common disorder is not well known, rarely tested for, and much less understood. It is estimated that over 62 million people in the U.S. alone suffer from digestive diseases, including LGS. Leakage of imperfectly digested proteins through a damaged intestinal lining is the root of many

Damaged Intestinal Lining

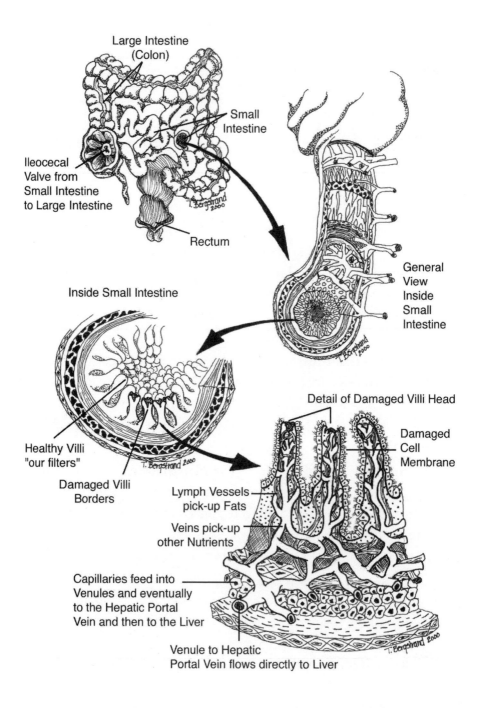

Large Intestine (Colon)

Small Intestine

Ileocecal Valve from Small Intestine to Large Intestine

Rectum

General View Inside Small Intestine

Inside Small Intestine

Detail of Damaged Villi Head

Damaged Cell Membrane

Healthy Villi "our filters"

Damaged Villi Borders

Lymph Vessels pick-up Fats

Veins pick-up other Nutrients

Capillaries feed into Venules and eventually to the Hepatic Portal Vein and then to the Liver

Venule to Hepatic Portal Vein flows directly to Liver

allergies and diseases. In a healthy gut, the intestinal lining is selectively porous to water and nutrients and normally resistant to most antigens and chemical toxins.

Some of the conditions associated with LGS are:
- Anaphylactic shock
- Candida (yeast overgrowth)
- Celiac disease
- Chemotherapy
- Chronic fatigue syndrome
- Chronic hepatitis
- Colitis
- Colon cancer
- Crohn's disease
- Environmental illness
- Fibromyalgia/Myofascial pain syndrome
- Food allergy, specific food intolerance
- *Giardia*
- Gout
- Inflammatory and infectious bowel diseases
- Inflammatory arthritis
- Irritable bowel syndrome
- Malnutrition
- Pancreatic dysfunction
- Parasitic involvement
- Skin conditions:
    eczema, psoriasis, dermatitis, hives

Hyper-permeability (abnormal leaking) may be the primary culprit in the biological role for the evolution of each disease, or it may be a secondary consequence, causing immune system activation (hypersensitivity), hepatic (liver) dysfunction, and pancreatic insufficiency.

The leakage of toxic substances from the intestine is usually controlled by the immune system. Eventually, the immune system gets overwhelmed. The overloaded system then allows toxins to leak and enter the liver, thus increasing the burden on the liver. When the liver cannot deal with the toxic overload, it flushes it back into the blood system, and all the body's alarm systems are triggered.

This is considered an attack to the immune system, so the circulatory system then pushes the toxins to the connective tissues and muscles. This is the body's way of storing the excess toxins in its inherent attempt to prevent major organ damage. If this condition continues, substances larger than particle size, such as disease-causing bacteria, potentially toxic molecules, and undigested food particles, are allowed to pass directly through the damaged cell membranes. This, in turn, sends them directly into the bloodstream, activating the alarm system and causing an allergic reaction. The body then releases histamines in response to cytokines, the alarm substances. These cytokines alert the lymphocytes (white blood cells) to fight the invading particles. Oxidants are produced in this response, causing irritation and inflammation. These symptoms are especially evident in allergies, arthritis, fibromyalgia, bowel disorders, and chronic fatigue. When the gut is not healthy, general health declines. *This inflammatory response is so far removed from the digestive system, the causes are usually overlooked.*

2

Autointoxication: How the Body POISONS Itself

Simply put, your plumbing system develops a leak, intestinal permeability, causing the intestinal materials and toxins to enter the body tissues, rather than being properly digested and carried through the intestines (small intestine and colon) to be eliminated. The leaked toxins then circulate to the liver, increasing its workload. The liver is now unable to neutralize the toxins or filter itself efficiently. If the liver can't deal with the toxic overload, it flushes it back into the blood (or stores it in soft connective tissues, manifested as inflammation) to deal with at a later time. If the toxins continue to leak through the intestinal mucosa, the liver never has the ability to detoxify what is already stored in soft connective tissues.

Compare this to shoving garbage down a kitchen sink. You figure a little garbage won't hurt. At first the water may run slower but it still flows (your body is still operating, but with impaired function, not often recognized until specific symptoms emerge). If you continue to pack the drain with garbage, the water and waste products will back up. Now you have garbage backing up in the kitchen sink and spilling onto the floor. This is similar to the backup occurring in your body. When food particles are not properly digested and eliminated they back up in the intestines and toxins leak into your body. Toxic matter gets stored throughout the body, as experienced in soft and connective tissue disorders like arthritis, fibromyalgia, and chronic fatigue. Inflammation occurs as the body attempts to deal with the stored toxins. This condition causes the eventual breakdown of the immune system.

The Role of the Large Intestine (Colon)

There are trillions of cells associated with the human body. Ninety percent are bacteria microflora microorganisms living in the large intestine, or colon. According to a leading expert on nutrition, Dr. Bernard Jensen, "Bacteria in our intestinal tract weigh nearly 3½ pounds, and are metabolically active." These bacterial microorganisms are essential to life, yet it's amazing how little is known or understood by traditional health-care providers about their powerful role.

It is now universally accepted that autointoxication, with its lack of adequate intestinal flora, is the underlying cause of an alarmingly large percentage of degenerative disorders and symptom complexes. The colonic micro-flora is a population of its own, taking up residence in your body. We know scientifically that a balance of good natural bacterial flora is imperative for health. Imbalances between the micro-flora and the body's operating systems can result in life-threatening implications from nutritional deficiencies, allergies, infection, impaired metabolism, toxicity, and cancer.

The Raging Fire within Us: Linking Inadequate Digestion and Autointoxication

When the digestive system is not operating to its full potential, improperly digested food molecules are not broken down sufficiently to be absorbed across the gut wall. These improperly digested food molecules are met with great enthusiasm by the "unfriendly" bacterial growth in the last section of the small intestine, the ileum. The unfriendly bacteria have a banquet on the food particles that are not adequately processed by the digestive system. Hence, they are fed just what they need to multiply at alarming rates.

Bacteria are a constant in the body, but are kept in balance in the healthy body by the predominance of "friendly" bacteria. The job of the friendly bacteria is to create an environment that restricts the growth or multiplication of unfriendly bacteria.

Lactobacilli and other coliform bacteria are the friendly bacteria, the same bacteria that promote the souring of milk. These bacteria must be greater in number than the unfriendly bacteria in order for the body to digest, assimilate, and eliminate. When this healthy process does not take place, due to the

Portal System connecting Colon to Liver via Veins and Lymph System

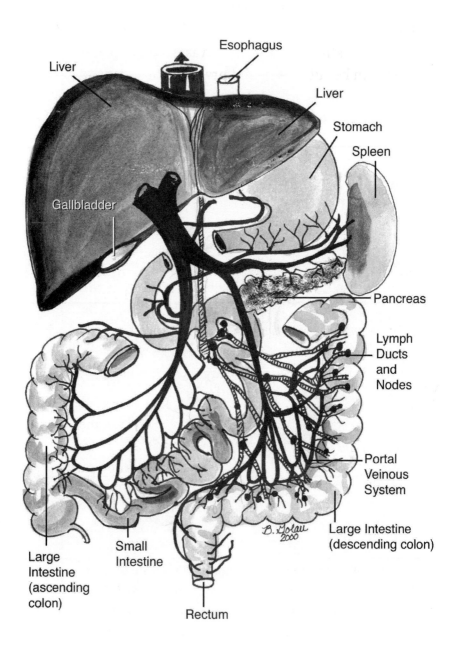

"bad guys" outnumbering the "good guys," putrefaction occurs. This process is a consequence of rotten food forming chemical toxins that are poisonous to the body.

If you stir a compost or waste material pile, there can be sufficient heat produced by the gasses to ignite a fire. In the case of our body, the toxic material ignites a series of symptom reactions as a consequence. We could say it "sets off the fire alarms" in the body's attempt to deal with the poisons. Our internal fire manifests as symptoms to warn us of impending metabolic burnout.

The chemicals produced by putrefaction are so poisonous they irritate the delicate lining of the colon. If this condition persists, it destroys the protective barrier keeping out the invading toxins. Damage from the chemical toxins is so destructive the colon walls become leaky and allow penetration through the damaged barrier into the lymphatic and circulatory systems especially through the hepatic portal vein. The more putrefaction, the more constipated the person. When the body becomes overwhelmed with toxins it can't handle, it becomes a raging fire on a path of self-destruction.

At this stage, the body is poisoning itself.

As the biological alarms for survival are triggered, the result is a breakdown of the immune system, resulting in numerous diseases, inflammation disorders, food allergies, allergic reactions, and

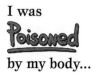

I was by my body...

eventual death. Death may be reported to be from a specific disease, such as liver or kidney failure. What are not usually investigated are the initial causes leading to the disease process in the first place.

3

Gut Reactions:
Symptoms of Leaky Gut

The following is a list of classic symptoms experienced with leaky gut syndrome (LGS). In most cases, leaky gut is the root cause often overlooked in the clinical diagnoses. Keep in mind that this condition is a syndrome; it stems from multiple causes.

Symptoms of Leaky Gut Syndrome:
- Abdominal pain
- Acute/chronic insomnia
- Anaphylactoid reactions
- Bloating/excessive gas
- Difficulty breathing
- Excessive anxiety or aggressiveness
- Fevers of unknown origin
- Gluten intolerance (celiac disease)
- Hemorrhoids
- Heartburn/acid reflux

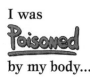
- Malnutrition
- Migraine headaches
- Multiple chemical sensitivities
- Muscle cramps
- Muscle pain
- Myofascial pain
- Mood swings
- Poor exercise tolerance
- Poor immunity
- Poor memory
- Recurrent bladder/urinary infection
- Recurrent vaginal infections
- Recurring skin rashes
- Sudden hair loss and nail changes
- Swollen lymph glands
- Sudden onset of food allergies
- Chronic constipation/diarrhea (dependence on laxatives)
- Liver dysfunction-pain or swelling/yellow tone to skin and eyes
- Brain fatigue

Autoimmune Response:
The Birth of Allergic Reactions

Allergies can be produced by an endless list of substances present in our food, water, and drugs, as well as in what we breathe, touch, and wear. Allergies are the body's reaction to antigens (foreign or unrecognized substances). When the body is in good natural health, it has the ability to deal with antigens as a normal course of function. Consequently, the one symptom of inflammatory and immune disorders is the formation of antibodies in response to the antigens. In LGS these materials leak across the intestinal wall and become antigens to our own tissues. As our body produces antibodies to attack them, it also attacks our tissues. It is suspected that this is how autoimmune diseases get their start. *The body is literally reacting to itself.* Rheumatoid arthritis, lupus, multiple sclerosis, thyroid disease, and many other debilitating conditions are fast becoming the ever-growing "incurable" diseases.

Rashes: More than Skin Deep

In my case, the rashes and blotches from leaky gut occurred only on the face and neck. However, many clients report a long history of skin disorders, including eczema, rosacea, and psoriasis.

It's been my experience that a skin disorder is the body's attempt to fight a foreign substance it does not have the mechanism to handle. In response to the invading antigen, inflammation occurs, as well as destruction of its own tissues. Any part of the body can be involved. In LGS, the recurrent rashes are connected as much to the body's ability to eliminate toxins as to the allergic antigen itself, as in multiple chemical sensitivities.

The skin is the body's largest organ. It is responsible for the greatest amount of detoxification; however, most people do not consider the skin an organ.

Gastrointestinal/Digestive System

The core of the digestive system is the gastrointestinal tract. The gastrointestinal (GI) tract is a hollow tube that begins at the mouth, where food enters the digestive system, and ends at the anus, where fecal waste products are expelled. Between the mouth and anus are the esophagus, stomach, small intestine, and large intestine. The vital organs of the liver, pancreas, and gallbladder support this diverse and essential tract. Collectively, these organs make up the digestive system.

The Work of the Digestive System

As food passes through the stomach by way of the mouth and esophagus, it enters the long, coiled tube of the small intestine.

The majority of absorption takes place in the small intestine. By the action of chewing, digestive juices are secreted and food is reduced to a liquid called chyme by the time it reaches the small intestine. Digestion of carbohydrates starts in the mouth with saliva. Proteins are broken down into short-chain fatty acids (the essential ingredients of protein formation) in the stomach. Further reduction of the chyme occurs until the molecules can be properly absorbed. Chyme entering through the pyloric valve from the stomach to the duodenum is highly acidic.

Gastrointestinal Digestive System

Mouth

Esophagus

Liver

Stomach

Transverse Colon

Gallbladder

Pancreas

Ascending Colon

Small Intestine

Anus

Descending Colon

It contains hydrochloric acid and enzymes, required to break down larger molecules into smaller substances. These fluids neutralize the acidic chyme from the stomach, raising the pH from 3 to almost 8 and creating an environment better suited to lipid and carbohydrate digestion. Special cells in the intestinal wall secrete substances that combine with juices flowing from the gallbladder (bile) and the pancreas, by way of the pancreatic duct, into the duodenum.

The small intestine absorbs nutrients through the cells of the villi, which acts like a strainer to protect the absorption of any foreign substances. The average adult has approximately two hundred square feet of surface in the small intestine. The small, filtered molecules can pass into the cell lining (villi) and are then absorbed by tiny blood capillaries and eventually end up in the hepatic (liver) portal vein, where they are carried to the liver and reduced even further. This demonstrates the connection between the destruction of the villi and liver stress.

Gastrointestinal Symptoms Associated with LGS:
- Abdominal cramps/spasms
- Abdominal extension
- Alternating bowel function
- Anal irritation
- Belching/burping
- Bloating
- Constipation
- Diarrhea

- Flatulence (gas)
- Heartburn/acid reflux
- Hunger pains
- Indigestion
- Itchy anus
- Reduced appetite

Constipation and Diarrhea: Essentially the Same Disorder

Symptoms of Constipation:
- Painful bowel movements due to hardness of the stool
- Inability to have a complete elimination
- Bloating and gas
- Tender or distended abdomen
- Feeling of sluggishness
- Hemorrhoids
- Indigestion
- Depression or anxiety

Drug or Substance-Induced Constipation in LGS and Related Disorders:
Usually constipation is brought on by drugs and substances including, but not limited to, the following,

- Codeine, or other high-potency pain medications
  (Example: Hydrocodone APAP)
- Antacids containing aluminum
  (Example: Prevacid)
- Iron supplementation

- Some narcotic drugs and antidepressants
  (Examples: Lorazepam, Trazodone,
  Alprazolam, Xanax)

Symptoms of Diarrhea:

- Frequent bowel movements of watery waste
  material
- Feeling like elimination is not quite complete
- Bloating and gas
- Tender or distended abdomen
- Feeling of sluggishness and fatigue
- Hemorrhoids
- Indigestion
- Depression or anxiety
- Rectal burning or itching

Causes of Diarrhea and Related Disorders

In addition to the causes of constipation, malab-
sorption syndromes and overgrowth of unfriendly
bacteria in the intestines may cause diarrhea.

People with chronic diarrhea believe their colon
is not constipated because they move their bowels
several times a day. Yes, their eliminations may not
be constipated or condensed, but the cause of the
diarrhea is usually linked to irritation of the colon.
The diarrhea occurs as waste accumulations adhere
to the walls of the colon, causing irritation from the
accumulation of stagnant waste with the accompanying overgrowth of bacteria and parasites. As the
inflammation progresses, the colon passageway becomes narrow, thus allowing mainly liquids to be
expelled and compounding the problem of waste

accumulation. Chronic diarrhea responds remark-
ably well to an effective colon-cleansing program.

Food Intolerance

Exactly when an allergic sensitivity occurs is
determined by as many diverse factors as the allergies, including length of time to exposure and extent
of damage from the allergen. Most clients had no
evidence of food sensitivities prior to LGS. However, some people report intolerance to certain foods
after taking prescription drug medications, with gut
symptoms occurring later. Eating allergic foods releases irritant substances into the gut, causing
inflammation. Therefore, the complex question in
leaky gut syndrome is: which came first, the LGS
or the food allergy?

Non-steroidal anti-inflammatory drugs (NSAIDs),
while in the bloodstream and body tissues, reduce
inflammation; when they reach the gastrointestinal
tract they become irritants and cause damage to the
intestinal lining. This, in turn, develops into a reduced capacity to deal with certain foods. The
protein component of the food is a major trigger.

➤ Flashback ➤

*In my case, I had no known allergies to any food or
substance other than monosodium glutamate
(MSG), a preservative used especially in Chinese
food. The MSG sensitivity manifested as migraine
headaches. After taking NSAIDs and developing
leaky gut syndrome, the biggest challenge for me
was the resulting food intolerances.*

Any food or substance can cause an allergic reaction. Excessive carbohydrate consumption and the following foods are the most common causes:

- Beef
- Eggs
- Gluten-containing foods
- Tree nuts (pecans, walnuts)
- Pork
- Shellfish
- Wheat
- Nightshade vegetables
  (potatoes, tomatoes, peppers)

- Corn
- Fish
- Milk
- Peanuts
- Refined sugar
- Soy

Multiple Chemical Sensitivity Syndrome (MCSS)

I've devoted an entire chapter (Chapter 4) to multiple chemical sensitivity syndrome, an environmental illness. In many cases, as in my own, this syndrome develops as a result of leaky gut and a compromised immune system. Until gut health is addressed, eliminating environmental allergens alone will not provide total wellness.

Acute/Chronic Insomnia

Sleep disturbances are caused by such a multitude of factors it would be impossible to discuss them all in this book. The following are some of the contributing causes of sleep disturbances related to LGS and gastrointestinal disorders.

Causes of sleep disturbances related to LGS:

- Parasites
- Dysbiosis
- *Candida*
- Environmental and food sensitivities
- Chronic fatigue syndrome
- Fibromyalgia and myofascial pain syndrome
- NSAIDs
- Steroidal drugs, such as cortisone and prednisone
- Autointoxication

➤Flashback➤

I had never experienced insomnia before. Yes, the occasional sleepless night would occur as a result of an overactive mind or stress, never lasting more than one or two nights. After my life-threatening accident, as described in Chapter 5: "How did I get this way?", and the prescription medications for pain and inflammation, insomnia set in. Medically, the insomnia was thrown in as part of the symptoms resulting from the recently diagnosed fibromyalgia. The insomnia became so acute I would encounter weeks without sleeping more than one or two hours a night, many nights not at all.

My internist became so concerned he consulted with other specialists, while also conducting extensive personal research, only to say "We don't know what else to do." He suggested prescribing a stronger sleep medication and changing the drug when that particular formula was no longer effective. After much frustration on his part and mine, he handed me a book written by a sleep specialist, suggesting several relaxation techniques and possibly enrolling in a sleep disorder clinic. I thanked him for his extra efforts and walked out of his office determined to find real answers to my symptoms. I am convinced the trigger was the NSAIDs, because it was the only medication I took for an extended period of time. Little did I suspect the long-term damage being caused to my liver and gut.

Sudden Hair Loss

It's been my experience, personally and professionally, that certain pain and anti-inflammatory drugs can be responsible for sudden hair loss. I advise anyone taking prescription medications to first identify the warnings or contraindications in the *Physician's Desk Reference* (PDR). The PDR is the "Bible" of prescription drugs, their use, and contraindications. It is available at your local library, doctor's office, bookstore, or pharmacy. The Internet also has specific information sites for most drugs. If you have any questions, seek the assistance of your pharmacist.

➤Flashback➤

Sudden hair loss occurred shortly after I took prescription NSAIDs. My hair was coming out in chunks. Eventually my hair had to be cut very

*short, and styled to "cover up" the bald areas.
This is a frightening experience, and one that can
be avoided by seeking natural alternatives for pain
and inflammation.*

Liver Pain and Swelling:
With a "Side Order" of Ribs

It is common for an LGS patient, or anyone
with liver inflammation, to experience pain in the
upper thoracic region, shoulder blade, neck, and
shoulders. The challenge, as in my case, lies in
correctly identifying the association of the liver and
ribs. As the liver attempts to deal with the toxins
released from the allergic responses of drug therapy
and autointoxication, it can swell and place pressure on many organs. As the following account
clearly describes, the liver's diverse functions connect the digestive system to every other system in
the body.

➤ Flashback ➤

*My original symptoms of pain were all right-
sided, involving my thoracic area, neck, shoulder
and arm. At times, the pain was unbearable.
Holding the steering wheel of my car or getting in
and out of a chair was more than I could tolerate.
No one could find an apparent cause. I kept
describing my pain as if "my rib was poking
through my shoulder blade from my back to my
chest."*

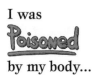
Finally, I was referred to Beata Golau, a thera-pist who incorporates specialized massage techniques in her therapeutic bodywork. She has also developed a course for health-care professionals. Her practice includes distinguished national and European clients and she is respectfully known as the "Rib Lady." The following is a synopsis of her findings during my therapy:

After an initial detailed consultation with Dr. Gilbère (Dr. G), I immediately suspected a misalignment of the first rib. Restrictions of the first rib are often the result of chronic contraction of the scalene muscles (Dr. G. humorously calls them scallions), which insert onto the rib. These powerful muscles gradually pull the rib up by as much as $1/4$ inch. There may be nerve irritation with local pain, as well as referred pain to the arm, neck, head, and chest. At the first session, I had her lie on the massage table thus gaining better access to the rib area to confirm my suspicion of rib-misalignment.

Since muscles move bone, I massaged the scalenes with a cross-fiber motion (a type of Myofacial Release Therapy) to reduce muscle tension. A firm, not hard, pressure is applied. Next I held the first ribs in place while she took a deep breath. The inhalation expands the rib cage, particularly the upper rib cage, creating room for the first rib to "go home" (which it does fairly easily). On the exhalation, the rib cage contracts around the re-seated rib and aligns. Often this procedure affords instant relief, as was the case with Dr. G.

The remainder of Dr. G's rib cage now needed atten-tion due to a right lower rib that felt like it was constantly poking. Upon examination, there were indeed two ribs over her liver area that had moved and were pressing

Drawing of Rib Cage
in Proportion to Nerves and Liver,
and Cause of Referred Pain

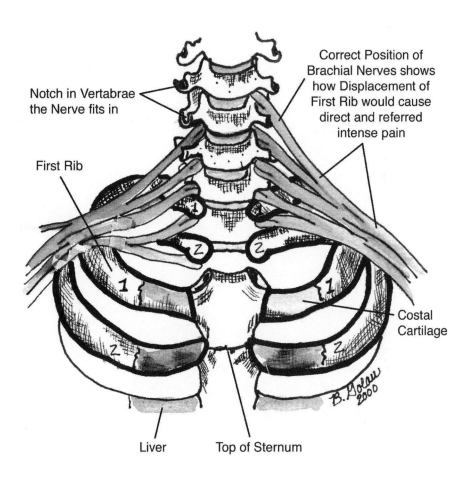

Correct Position of
Brachial Nerves shows
how Displacement of
First Rib would cause
direct and referred
intense pain

Notch in Vertabrae
the Nerve fits in

First Rib

Costal
Cartilage

Liver   Top of Sternum

against one another. With a similar deep breath technique, the ribs realigned, relieving the symptom of pressure and poking.

In the beginning, Dr. G and I believed we found the cause of her pain, misalignment and restrictions from muscle tension. Much to our surprise, we soon learned there was a direct correlation between liver inflammation and the misalignment of her ribs. It became evident that when muscles expanded as a direct response to the inflammation of the liver, it caused contractions that resulted in the ribs being pulled out of alignment. Eventually, when her liver inflammation was under control, so were the ribs and the associated pain.

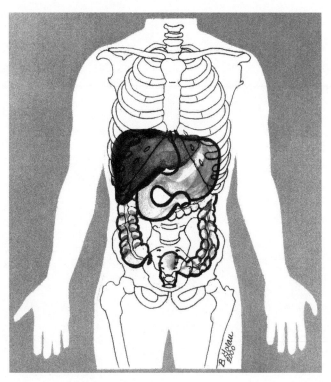

Ribcage in relationship to liver and large intestine

It is now evident that my liver involvement was a result of the prescription pain medications and NSAIDs. Most of my clients with a history of pain medications, steroidal drug therapy, or NSAIDs manifest similar symptoms, often undiagnosed by traditional methods. The majority consulted with several health-care professionals (some as many as ten) without permanent improvement. It is my intent that my example will assist clients and their health-care professionals to look at the symptoms with different lenses, adding clarity to the functional cause. Yes, hindsight is 20/20. Had I been able to pinpoint the cause of my initial intense pain, it would not have become necessary to take the pain medications or NSAIDs, which opened the way for the leaky gut and the resulting multiple chemical sensitivities.

Brain Fog: Your Mind is Writing Checks Your Body Can't Cash

Dysbiosis (unbalanced intestinal micro-flora) is a condition resulting from the prolific enzymatic activity of the intestinal lining. In an unbalanced environment, indigenous bacteria not only make vitamins (like Vitamin K) and destroy toxins, but they also destroy vitamins (like Vitamin B-12) and make toxins. Some by-products of bacterial activity, such as ammonia, hinder normal brain function. When absorbed into the body, the liver must remove these dangerous by-products. When the liver is not able to neutralize these substances, the results can be "foggy thinking." Brain fog, depression, attention deficit, and aggressive personality disorders are often linked to dysbiosis or systemic yeast overgrowth (described in detail in Chapter 5).

Anaphylactic Shock: Difficulty Swallowing

Anaphylactic shock is a life-threatening condition clinically known as anaphylaxis. The word anaphylactic means it has a relationship to a substance causing the shock (reaction). The term anaphylaxis refers to a hypersensitivity resulting from contact to the reactive substance.

During anaphylactic reactions people may feel uneasy and develop palpitations, tingling, itchy and flushed skin, throbbing heat in the ears, coughing, sneezing, hives, swelling, or increased difficulty breathing caused by asthma or closing off of the windpipe. Cardiovascular collapse can occur without respiratory symptoms. Usually an episode involves either respiratory or cardiovascular symptoms, not both, and the person has the same pattern of symptoms in subsequent episodes.

Anaphylactic reactions can cause a sudden drop of blood pressure and may lead to dizziness. The reaction may progress so rapidly it can lead to collapse, convulsions, loss of bladder control, unconsciousness, or stroke within one to two minutes. Anaphylaxis may prove fatal unless immediate emergency treatment is given. *(The Merck Manual of Medical Information, 1997.)*

In leaky gut syndrome, the causes of anaphylactic reactions become complicated. A reaction to a specific food is blamed solely on the food, and seldom linked to a medication or environmental exposure from hours, days, or months earlier. In my case, anti-inflammatory medications caused leaky gut, the leaky gut caused food allergies, and the overworked immune system triggered multiple chemical sensitivities.

➤Flashback◄

My first experience with throat-closure appeared after taking NSAIDs. Subsequently, anaphylactic reactions resulted after eating specific foods, as well as from having an empty stomach. My body began reacting to itself. In addition, as my immune system became overworked and less able to process toxins, I began to experience anaphylaxis when exposed to chemicals. Now I had the added challenge of multiple chemical sensitivities. I was forced to eliminate everything possible in my home and office that wasn't natural.

Not all people with digestive disorders and leaky gut syndrome develop severe allergic reactions, but most do. People with food allergies may react violently to eating even tiny amounts of the offending food. As an example, stirring a food that triggers an allergic response, then using the same utensil to stir a tolerated food, can cause a reaction. The small amount of offending food remaining on the utensil may never be suspected as a reaction trigger. To further complicate the syndrome, many people react to certain foods because the weakened digestive system lacks an enzyme necessary for digesting that specific food group.

Food additives are a large contributor to adverse allergic reactions and anaphylaxis. Major contributors to food responses are monosodium glutamate (MSG), food preservatives such as sulfites, artificial sweeteners, and dyes. Chemicals found in many products such as candles, soft drinks, and clothing, to mention a few, add to the complex reactions associated with multiple chemical sensitivity (see Chapter 4).

Heartburn/Acid Reflux

Heartburn (also called "acid stomach") is a burning pain in the stomach that spreads across the chest. The glands of the stomach produce a number of substances, including hydrochloric acid and various food digesting enzymes. When the acid backs up into the esophagus, heartburn results. It generally occurs after a meal and especially when lying down. It can result in gastro-esophageal reflux (GERD), a common disorder occurring when the stomach's contents back up into the esophagus. Food allergies, toxic colon, and lack of enzymes are contributing factors.

A faulty digestive and elimination system allows fermentation of food in the stomach and colon. Fermentation of food in the colon produces hydrogen methane and carbon dioxide that feed bacteria and cause gas, bloating, and eventually LGS. This overgrowth of unfriendly intestinal flora then becomes dysbiosis.

Antacids, including such drugs as Prevacid, Tagamet (cimetidine), and Zantac (ranitidine), are the common conventional treatment. These treatments are generally effective based on the theory that the pain of indigestion and heartburn is due to excess stomach acid. In 1990, clinical studies showed that antacids were of no real benefit for the majority of patients with heartburn. While they may provide some immediate relief, they don't address the underlying causes. Granted, the use of antacids increases the production of hydrochloric acid by the parietal cells breaking down food for digestion. However, the cells producing hydrochloric acid become so overworked they ultimately produce less and less hydrochloric acid.

Another side effect of antacids is their ability to decrease protein-digesting enzymes, such as protease, already deficient in people with digestive disorders. Antacids are alkaloid buffers that neutralize acids and raise pH. Proteases, such as pepsin, require low pH environments for effectiveness. The antacid does not destroy the enzyme; it destroys the environment for effectiveness. For example, freezing does not destroy water, but only reduces its ability to flow.

Dehydration/Mineral Loss

In intestinal disorders, particularly leaky gut, there is usually a deficiency of minerals.

➤Flashback ➤

At the onset of my leaky gut, I had severe muscle cramps, commonly known as "charley horses," in the calves of my leg. There were many nights I would abruptly sit up in bed and scream with intolerable cramps. An additional symptom was muscle pain and coldness in my legs. It felt as if I had an I.V. of ice water running through my legs. A patient with fibromyalgia or leaky gut understands the type of pain I'm describing. The pain is deep-seated within the muscles and generally chronic, especially late in the day and at night. It's a feeling of "hurting and soreness all over" with no visible evidence! Once I started mineral replacement, the symptoms vanished.

See "Supplementing Minerals 'My Whey'" in Chapter 7 for details on mineral supplementation.

4

Multiple Chemical Sensitivity Syndrome (MCSS) is Environmental Illness (EI)

As if having leaky gut with the resulting food allergies isn't enough, multiple chemical sensitivity syndrome (MCSS), an environmental illness (EI), usually develops as well. MCSS is marked by *multiple symptoms in multiple organ systems* (usually the neurological, immune, respiratory, skin, gastrointestinal, and musculoskeletal). MCSS is a side effect of a weakened immune system that is not able to neutralize toxins in a toxic world.

MCSS is an adverse reaction to toxic chemicals in air, food, or water at concentrations generally considered harmless to the healthy population. However, when a healthy body is repeatedly exposed to toxic chemicals, the body develops a decreased tolerance. The immune system becomes overburdened, leading to autoimmune disorders. When a person with a compromised immune system is exposed to toxic chemicals, *the sick get sicker,* and may even die from the resulting reaction.

People with MCSS manifest acute sensitivity from natural gas fumes, gasoline, car exhaust, dyes and to chemicals in fabrics, clothes and fabrics containing synthetics, carpets, cleaning materials, phenolated compounds, perfumes, and smoke from cigarettes or other sources, to mention a few.

After World War II, a new generation of chemicals was synthesized, including pesticides, synthetic fragrances, cleaning products, food preservatives and coloring, and detergents, mostly petrochemicals (petroleum based) and *very toxic to humans.* I call them "baby boomer chemicals." These chemicals were, and still are, considered "safe, until proven toxic." Dr. Theron G. Randolph, then a professor at Northwestern University, first described MCSS in the 1950s, when MCSS was considered the 20th Century Disease. As a side effect of our modern industrialized society, we are all participants in a global chemical experiment, and it's making millions of us very sick.

In the past, coal miners didn't need high-tech equipment to measure air quality. They simply took a caged canary into the mine with them; if the bird stopped singing or died, the air was toxic and they got out. People with MCSS are the human canaries of the 21st century, warning that the air in our homes, offices, and environment is toxic. If those of us with MCSS continue to be exposed to toxic chemicals, we can become dead canaries, rather than the wounded canaries serving as early-warning systems through our allergic reactions.

According to studies conducted by the California Department of Health in 1995 and published in *Multiple Chemical Sensitivity Research Reports,* 17-34 percent of Americans report symptoms of chemical sensitivity. The studies also show that two-thirds of patients with MCSS have been diagnosed with chronic fatigue syndrome and fibromyalgia. Furthermore, it is estimated that 50 percent of office visits in general practice today are related to complaints of food and environmental allergies.

As the gut heals, and we minimize or eliminate exposure to toxic substances and support the body's detoxification, digestion, assimilation, and elimination, the symptoms of fibromyalgia, chronic fatigue, and MCSS are dramatically reduced or eliminated. Reduction of toxic exposure facilitates healing by reducing the body's total toxic load. The dramatic improvement of secondary symptoms adds support to my belief that these syndromes have a "gut cause."

Intolerance vs. Allergic Reaction

Allergies occur at any stage in life and include essentially all disorders of the immune system that involve a heightened sensitivity to substances. The distinction between being allergic to something and simply having a poor tolerance is extremely important. In any case, you *must* avoid the substance. Especially in leaky gut and multiple chemical sensitivity syndromes, as with any diseases that compromise the immune system, the continued or total accumulated exposure (TAE) may turn from intolerance to a life-threatening reaction. For example, if you are intolerant of penicillin, the symptoms may be diarrhea. However, if you are allergic to it, the reaction may kill you. Today, it is estimated that over eight hundred deaths occur every year from a penicillin reaction that leads to anaphylaxis, and that accounts for just one substance.

Symptoms of MCSS/EI

The symptoms of MCSS/EI generally start out slowly. At first you may notice an increased sensitivity to environmental smoke or fragrances. It starts out simply: being extra sensitive while walking by a perfume counter, candle department, or a recently cleaned room. You may first experience a headache, itchy eyes or skin. The exhaust from cars may now precipitate a rash, shortness of breath, or the immediate need for fresh air. Chemicals such as hair spray, hair color, permanent waves, deodorant, glass and bathroom cleaner, fingernail polish and remover, or nonstick cooking spray all bring on some type of reaction. Pesticides used on a lawn may trigger a reaction and, at first, may be brushed off as hay fever or seasonal allergies. Most people with MCSS/EI manifest escalating intolerance to loud noises, bright lights, and extremes of heat and cold. It *appears* that we suddenly react to a variety of inhalants, chemicals, and mold, not evident before developing leaky gut.

There are two main types of allergic/hypersensitive responses.

Type One Allergic Response

Type One is an immediate-onset allergy. This is the mechanism that binds immunoglobulin E (IgE) antibodies to a specific antigen (a food or inhalant). When white blood cells are sensitized to produce the specific IgE antibodies and then contact the specific antigen, the cells, in defense, release powerful substances. When produced in excess, these substances are destructive and inflammatory, produce symptoms usually within thirty minutes, and damage normal tissues. These substances include lysosomal enzymes, histamine, toxic oxygen radicals, arachidonic acid, leukotriences, kinin and bradykinin-like substances, and dehydroascorbic acid. The lysosomal enzymes literally digest and destroy tissue. Histamine causes leakage from capillaries, producing swelling, constriction of bronchioles, excessive mucus production, and much more.

Environmental allergens can be anything you breathe or touch, such as pollen, perfume, chemicals, or smoke. The following is a limited list of symptoms resulting from exposure to the excessive release of inflammatory substances.

Responses to Environmental Allergens:
- Accelerated response to heat
- Anaphylactic shock
- Anxiety or panic attacks
- Asthma attacks

- Chills
- Difficulty breathing
- Edema (swelling)
- Heart irregularities
- Hives/rashes
- Intestinal spasms
- Itchy eyes
- Memory loss
- Mood swings (depression, extreme highs and lows)
- Muscle aches or cramping
- Nasal discharge/post-nasal drip
- Sensitivity to weather changes
- Sinus congestion
- Sudden acute headaches
- Tingling or numbness on tongue or lips

Type Two Allergic Response

These reactions are considered non-IgE reactions and therefore are not a true allergy, but produce an allergy-like response. These reactions involve IgG antibodies, IgG immune complexes, IgM and IgA antibodies, and cellular T-lymphocyte mediated responses. These responses all have delayed onset of symptoms, usually forty-eight to seventy-two hours or more, after eating the allergic food or exposure to airborne allergen and are usually the most difficult to specifically diagnose.

Type Two responses are as destructive as Type One and possibly more significant because of the masked underlying culprit contributing to serious chronic and autoimmune diseases. The next time you feel spacey, dopey, or unable to concentrate, retrace the exposures of the previous few days. For many people with leaky gut, fibromyalgia, chronic fatigue, and MCSS, the delayed symptoms accelerate the generalized muscle pain and fatigue, making it harder to identify the culprit. When traditional drug therapies continue to treat symptoms and not causes, the sick get sicker. If you suspect delayed onset of symptoms, consider the following:

Were You:

- In a room with new carpet or rugs?
- In a new or recently remodeled building?
- Exposed to a new computer, copier, or electronic equipment?
- Exposed to new paint or varnishes?
- On a recently fertilized lawn or golf course?
- In a hardware, automotive, or paint store?
- Recently in a dry cleaning establishment?
- In a barber or beauty salon?

Do You:

- Have new furniture (wood or upholstered)?
- Have new draperies or synthetic window coverings?
- Microwave food in plastic containers, especially Styrofoam?
- Have a new computer?
- Have a new electric stove?

Did you:

- Visit a hospital or medical building?
- Purchase a new synthetic pillow, mattress pad, or blanket?
- Polish your shoes indoors?
- Spend time in a moldy basement or building?
- Have recent exposure to natural gas or propane appliances?
- Recently use a self-cleaning oven?

Have you:

- Visited a fabric department or fabric store?
- Slept on new, unwashed bedding?
- Recently cleaned the interior of your car?
- Recently purchased a vehicle?

My intent in relating this information connecting MCSS and leaky gut is to promote awareness of the myriad causes of allergic reactions. My goal is to help you take control of your life, heal your immune system, and again enjoy quality of life and function in society.

Effects of MCSS/EI

The damage to the detoxification system, especially the liver and lymphatics, may eventually extend to all body systems because they are interdependent. If the liver is unable to detoxify (break down) and use a chemical, the chemical ends up floating around the circulatory system, available to every cell. If damage occurs in the musculoskeletal system, symptoms may result in chronic pain and weakness, as experienced in fibromyalgia and chronic fatigue. If damage occurs in the nervous system, symptoms may include depression, anxiety, brain fog, and feeling "spacey." If the damage is in the respiratory system, the symptoms may propel a sudden onset of acute asthma or chronic bronchitis.

Life with MCSS/EI Takes on a New Meaning

A combination of food and environmental sensitivities alters a life-style like no one can imagine, unless actually experienced. Any environment beyond our control becomes a huge risk factor until the immune system detoxifies and repairs. People facing these challenges can get very discouraged. A new set of symptoms can emerge weekly, daily, even hourly.

A stroll in a shopping mall, attending worship services, flying, a doctor's office visit, a trip to the hairdresser, or having a repair-person come to your home is no longer predictable. One way to eliminate or drastically reduce your exposure is to wear a mask with a charcoal filter. I wore several styles of heavy masks that were uncomfortable and unsightly, until I discovered a line made by "I can breathe". They contain a disposable charcoal filter and have allowed me to travel, shop and resume quality of life. People actually stop me in airports and public places asking me where to get one. I use it when I go outdoors during the farmers' field burning season

...ple
Chemical
Sensitivity
Syndrome
(MCSS) is
Environmental
Illness (EI)

51

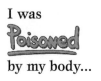
52

and it completely protects me. They are so small and lightweight they fit in the palm of your hand and are as flexible as a handkerchief (see product resources). I now have clients purchasing them for all their airline travel, even those without MCS. It protects them from the barrage of germs, pesticides and germicides in a space with re-circulated air. It allows them to arrive at their destination without travelers "flu".

Stress: Adding Fuel to the Fire

Seemingly unrelated exposures and events can trigger symptoms. Prior to developing leaky gut, a stressful situation might have been just that, a situation. However, now the added component of toxic environmental exposure can cause a myriad of symptoms, including rashes and swelling of the throat. This reaction occurs because stress releases abnormal amounts of toxins and the body system is already overloaded in coping with leaky gut syndrome and the resulting disorders.

The connection between the mind and the immune system is an important one. This does *not* mean the immune system's reaction is "psychological." In allergic responses to emotional stress, the immune system responds by activating protective mechanisms (reactions) to warn of impending danger.

According to Dr. Hans Selye, pioneer in studies of the physical effects of stress, the initial changes taking place in reaction to stress (a surge of adrenaline, increased heart rate, rash) are designed to help you escape a dangerous situation. The situation may be social, such as anger or fear, or physical, such as avoiding or being a participant in an accident. Fear and anger act on the autonomic nervous system, controlling the functions of internal organs, blood components, and lymph vessels. In severe cases, emotional stress can bring on anaphylaxis, the systemic allergic reaction where airways swell and close; the person may go into shock or die.

➤Flashback ◀

I encountered interpersonal situations that became so challenging that I had to completely discontinue communication with the individuals. The situation is especially difficult when it involves family members. We need people we care about to understand or at least be emotionally supportive, and it's heartbreaking when they aren't. To the individuals pushing my "stress" buttons, my decision to eliminate stressful situations by refusing to engage in further confrontations appeared to be "selfish" and "self-serving." It was! Selfish, because I chose to take whatever measures were necessary for survival. Yes, self-serving, because I was determined to conquer this debilitating disorder, help others as a result of my experience, and take back control of my life and health.

Different Day, Different Symptom

Because individuals are biochemically different, there are tremendous individual variations in the response to chemical allergens. Since the environment is always changing, so are the reactions. Substances may cause a reaction one day and not another. Total accumulated exposure (TAE), as I've named it, creates a decreased tolerance. Therefore, the more we're exposed to allergens, the less we can tolerate.

No two people will exhibit the same reaction to environmental conditions. Environmental illness can be difficult to diagnose because of the varied symptoms. Routine blood tests frequently indicate that no problem exists. Fortunately, there are more and more medical and health-care professionals who *do* recognize that EI usually has a gut cause. Many clients are treated with drugs for digestive disorders, only to be given more drugs when multiple chemical sensitivities develop. This emphasizes the practice of symptom-care, instead of health-care. Yes, drugs save lives (including my own) but, in my opinion, they should be used as urgent care, not symptom maintenance, and then only until root causes are identified and natural solutions initiated.

The key to wellness lies in minimizing and reversing damage to body systems by avoiding or limiting continued exposure to toxic environments. In today's toxic environment everybody *appears* fated to suffer some form of EI. The only way to effect positive changes is through education and personal responsibility. Each person's total accumulated exposure is like a volcano, building excessive gasses in the gastrointestinal tract, waiting to erupt with an allergic response. At first exposure, we may develop minor allergies. Eventually, the immune system is overworked, as in leaky gut, and the allergies become acute.

Your Internal Toxic Tocsin (ITT)

When people become sensitized to chemicals, they will react at levels not detectable by others. I refer to this as the "internal toxic tocsin (ITT)." A tocsin, according to Webster's, is an "alarm or signal." The word originated from *tocar,* meaning to touch or ring a bell. Just as a smoke detector is triggered by smoke as a warning of impending danger, your ITT is the body's alarm system signaling toxic overload, as experienced in an allergic response.

Life is no longer ordinary, even though on the outside we may *appear* just fine (unless you're like I was, yellow with jaundice, swollen with rashes, and suddenly fifty pounds lighter). If someone has a visible challenge (broken limb or paralysis), the seriousness leaves little to be questioned. If a person is challenged with multiple syndromes (leaky gut, fibromyalgia, chronic fatigue, multiple chemical sensitivities) the effects are not immediately evident to the observer, and if they are, they occur during the reaction and then visibly disappear. In some people, the resulting skin disorders are always present but in varying degrees. The victim must alert others that internal swelling and restricted breathing is occurring (unless they're unable to speak while gasping for air and grabbing the throat). If you ever witness someone experiencing an anaphylactic reaction, you will never forget it!

Your ITT may also respond by producing excessive mucus, nasal congestion, bronchial constriction, itching, or headache. These alarms, although not immediately as serious, are still an alarm.

For me, as for millions with environmental illness, drastic measures must be taken to control toxic exposure; these measures are essential for us to live, function, and restore health.

➤Flashback◄

For several months, my housemate and I detected strong chemical odors penetrating the house late at night. It was an inconvenience; however, the implications of long-term effects were not immediately evident. It is not unusual in a rural farm area to experience heavy smoke from field and trash burning, so we dismissed it as a seasonal nuisance that would eventually go away.

At first, our symptoms were minor, a slight headache and sore throat. Then, every time the smell was detected, we would develop headaches, nasal congestion, and excessive mucous (indicating decreased tolerance).

Shortly after my diagnosis of leaky gut, I experienced my first frightening reaction to environmental exposure. Since the development of leaky gut, I had first-hand experience with anaphylactic reactions from foods not tolerated, but not from an environmental allergen. One evening I was awakened by an especially strong toxic odor penetrating the open window in my bedroom. Within ten minutes, my face began to swell and itch, I developed a pounding frontal headache, and my throat began to swell. I knew something extremely toxic was burning; the smell was the same as in the past, only now much stronger. The only clues: a neighbor still burned his trash, the smell was always late at night, and the odor was stronger on cloudy nights. That evening, after assisting me through the anaphylactic reaction, my housemate followed the toxic smell. Indeed, a neighbor was burning trash. To make matters worse, upon investigation we found evidence of burned plastics and automobile oil filters. The individual acknowledged responsibility and stopped burning. However, the exposure triggered serious allergic reactions to environmental allergens not previously experienced.

A client relayed another case of potentially life-threatening toxic exposure caused by an individual insensitive to implications of their actions: During a commercial flight, a woman passenger was removing her nail polish. Many nail-polish removers

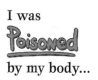
and nail polish products contain toluene, a known carcinogen, as well as other toxic chemicals like acetone. The use of this substance in an enclosed airplane cabin with re-circulating air makes this situation very dangerous. The woman passenger was annoyed when asked, by my client, to refrain from using the substance because of its toxic nature and the risk posed to passengers and crew, especially those with multiple chemical sensitivities.

This was a seemingly innocent act with the potential for devastating consequences. It is alarming to imagine the unsuspecting pollutants inhaled from an airborne toxin during a routine airplane flight. What should be of equal concern is that this type of hazard *can* be completely avoided, if people take responsibility for the substances they use and the potential hazards posed to people and the environment. As more and more people react to environmental pollutants, education is the master key to prevention. Knowledge is power, power to protect and heal ourselves and the environment through education. The power to eliminate toxic pollutants begins when consumers refuse to buy or use products that are not natural. In this way we *do* make a difference, one person at a time.

After relating the above story to another client, she described a specific incident experienced with nail polish remover, confirming its level of toxicity. She was using nail polish remover in her bathroom, and it activated the carbon monoxide detector. The incident initially peaked her concern, but was soon forgotten until we entered into a discussion about my increasing sensitivities to commonly used highly toxic chemicals. Our conversation stirred my insatiable curiosity. I asked a science teacher to conduct the same test with another brand of nail-polish remover and, again, the carbon monoxide detector was activated! When I investigated *just one* of the many toxic ingredients contained in the polish remover, toluene, I found that it's no wonder the detector was activated. Toluene is a liquid hydrocarbon (C_7H_8), resembles benzene, is flammable, is a toxic solvent, and is used as an anti-knock additive in gasoline. Hydrocarbon is a constituent present in petroleum, natural gas, and coal. I rest my case for the seriousness of generalized toxic exposure to chemicals like toluene, especially in a public area in an enclosed space with recirculating air. I hope this example will raise individual awareness and responsibility to the potential risks posed by substances that we routinely use.

The following account chronicles my personal experience with recirculating air.

➤ Flashback ◄

I was scheduled for my routine dental cleaning in an office I had been in many times within the past several years. On this particular visit, and after developing leaky gut syndrome and MCSS/EI, I entered the reception area, announced my arrival, and read a magazine while waiting to be called for my appointment.

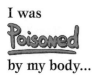
Within a few minutes my face was itching and turning red. I also developed a frontal headache. When I relayed my symptoms to the hygienist, she commented that she and several staff members were recently experiencing symptoms of headaches and red, irritated eyes. No new equipment or dental products were in the dental office. She suspected that something toxic was circulating from within the medical building. We decided to proceed with the dental cleaning, since I had traveled two hours and it would be months before I could be rescheduled. The hygienist was not finished when I exclaimed, "I have to get out of here."

By the time I left, my eyes looked as if they were painted red, my throat felt as if it was sandpapered, and a rash was progressing down my neck as the headache continued to pound. After leaving the building, I walked in the fresh winter air and the acute symptoms subsided. The eye redness disappeared within a couple of hours, but the headache and sore throat continued. Within three days, I had lumps the size of golf balls on my neck; my lymph system was swollen from dealing with the extraordinary load of toxins. The lingering effects from the exposure in the dental office building continued for three weeks, along with a sore throat, muscle pain and fatigue. I was a "lucky canary"; I fled the building, just in the nick of time.

*Chemical
Sensitivity
Syndrome
(MCSS) is
Environmental
Illness (EI)*

61

There was definitely something very toxic circulating in the building. The office is located in a large multi-use medical facility and the ventilation system is interconnected. The exact source of the pollutant is difficult to detect. My experience added validity to the concerns and symptoms of the employees and prompted a search for the toxic origin. I became the internal toxic tocsin, an early warning of danger lingering in the air. In this instance, I became the "wounded canary" and fortunately not the dead one.

Digging Your Teeth into
Multiple Chemical Sensitivities

During the 1960s and 70s I worked in dentistry. I had all the amalgam (silver) fillings and other restorations removed and replaced by gold, acrylic, or a combination of alloy and porcelain. No one suspected that years later the alloys used in dental restorations would be found detrimental to health. In individuals with weakened immune systems, like LGS and MCSS/EI, the exposure to alloys can cause an array of symptoms, some serious.

After developing leaky gut, I developed gingivitis, an inflammation of the gums. This was not surprising, because oral health is one of the first indicators of a weakened immune system and poor nutrition. The gums were so sensitive it was torture to brush, much less use toothpaste. I finally resorted to baking soda and salt, which still caused discomfort, but to a lesser degree. Attempts by my dentist, hygienist, and me to eliminate the inflammation were unsuccessful. Finally, when my leaky gut improved substantially, so did the inflammation. However, there were two teeth that were chronically inflamed. The surrounding tissue was bright red, swollen, and bled from the slightest pressure.

The two teeth involved were my upper cuspids (eye teeth). They were restored in 1966 using porcelain fused to metal. The metal used was an alloy base containing titanium; the porcelain was baked over the crown cast of metal. At the time of restoration, this type of porcelain crown was the best. Since I worked in the office that prepared and made the crowns, I discussed my restorative options with the dentist and the dental lab technician. I decided on titanium, since it was the dental metal of choice for restorative dentistry in the 60s. I recall joking about the potential of titanium setting off metal detectors.

Finally, as my multiple chemical sensitivities escalated, my local dentist expressed concern for potential sensitivity to the alloy used in this type of crown. I again "dug my teeth in" and researched the use of dental alloys containing titanium. What I found is alarming. According to a study conducted by *Biomedical Engineering News,* "the integrity of restorative dentistry devices containing titanium may be compromised because of the galvanic corrosion problem." The study was designed to measure direct galvanic or coupled corrosion properties of dental restorative and implant materials with titanium. Their testing monitored continuous corrosion potential in conjunction with zero-resistance ammetry. In essence, dental work consisting of titanium could be rusting away!

I relate my personal experience, and the results of the study, to illustrate the potential chemical hazard and biochemical reaction of restorative dental work, particularly in persons with MCSS/EI. If you have restorative dentistry and MCSS/EI, consult with a dentist who is knowledgeable in dealing with chemical sensitivities and willing to work with your health-care provider. I'm extremely fortunate to have a dentist who "dug" for the cause of my inflammation. The next challenge was finding a replacement for the crown, and the cementing material, with a lower potential for reaction.

Isn't it unfortunate that our beautiful restorative dental work has the potential to take a "bite" out of our health?

Alert:

Be sure your dentist is prepared to administer anesthetics that contain *no preservatives*. This is an area often overlooked, with serious consequences. If you have problems with the preservative-free anesthetic, ask your dentist about safe options for anesthesia (such as nitrous oxide or acupuncture). Don't assume he's prepared; discuss your needs with the dentist, not a staff member. Chemical reactions can be life threatening, and require serious precautions. Don't risk misinterpretation by a third party. Until your body repairs, and your tolerance to foreign chemicals lessen, your trip to the dental office will not be the same. You may be confronted with new sensitivities, not evident until you experience a chemical reaction. It would be impossible to predict the outcome of exposure to the many chemicals used in any medical facility, and dentistry is no exception. Remember to consult with your dentist about the seriousness of your sensitivities *before* you need to make the trip to the dental office. Even lingering chemicals in the air can trigger a reaction. It is best to schedule an appointment first thing in the morning, to reduce exposure to a daily buildup of substances. Be sure your dentist and you are both prepared.

➤ Flashback ➤

After developing LGS and MCSS/EI, my dentist took extraordinary steps to prevent a reaction. Fortunately, he has experience in dealing with MCSS/EI and incorporates a wholistic approach in his practice. Neither one of us knew what to expect. He protected my face from direct contact to latex, scheduled my appointment first thing in the morning, and used minimum local anesthetic. During my dental appointment, everything was fine; I had no immediate reaction. Within an hour of returning home, I developed a pounding headache. At first, I dismissed the symptom as stress-related. As the day and evening progressed, the headache intensified and became acute. I felt as if my brain was swollen and my scalp bruised. The next day I had extreme exhaustion. I contacted my dentist, who had already called after office hours to check on me, and I reported the escalating headache. Similar symptoms had been experienced in patients with MCSS/EI. He believed the cause was the preservative in the local anesthetic. The headache finally disappeared after two days, while lingering fatigue and light-headedness lasted several more days. For my subsequent dental work, my dentist special-ordered local anesthetic without preservatives to reduce the risk of reacting. I had no reaction to the preservative-free anesthetic.

Other Lessons Learned

My struggle continues with multiple chemical sensitivities, comprised of daily improvements and challenges with an illness that changes every aspect of one's life *forever*. In my forthcoming books about MCSS/EI, I share advice chronicling my personal journey to wellness, scientific research, solutions and lessons learned. They provide a comprehensive resource from a wholistic approach, offering tangible prevention and relief from environmental illness.

After extensive research and personal experience with chemical reactions, I discovered the following two products that provided me with non-toxic options for cleaning and personal care.

I was reacting to every cleaning product imaginable until I was introduced to Green 4 Clean manufactured by IPAX Cleanogel, Inc. This product is so safe and environmentally conscious that the Environmental Illness Society of Canada (EISC) has endorsed it. It's a highly concentrated liquid that's tolerated by the majority of people afflicted with MCS. Green 4 Kleen is:

- 100% Water soluable ▪ Contains No VOC's
- 100% Environmentally Safe ▪ No Fumes or Odors
- Non-Toxic ▪ Non-Flammable ▪ Non-Corrosive
- Contains No Mineral Spirits, Petroleum, Solvents
- Non-Alkali ▪ Contains No Phosphates
- 100% Active Ingredients ▪ Removes and Inhibits Mold
- Will Not Harm People, Animals or Plants
- Leaves a Surgically Clean Surface
- Complies with all E.P.A., U.S.D.A., and MIOSHA Regulations
- Contains No Caustics or Corrosives

I use this product for all my cleaning: carpet, laundry, baths, painted surfaces, wood floors, tile, car maintenance, kitchen, degreaser, stainless, sealed wood. It can be used on any surface where water is safe (see product reference).

I was also reacting to shampoos, moisture creams, hormone replacement creams, facial and body cleansers. I discovered a company that manufacturers a certified organic line including all the products mentioned above. The company is Organic Excellence (see product reference). None of the skin care products have fragrance, and the hair care products have an organic "hint" of mint. They do NOT contain: Sodium Lauryl Sulfate, Olefin Sulfonate, Propylene Glycol, Mureth Sulfate, Ammonium Lauryl Sulfate or derivatives of Lauryl Alcohol.

5

How Did I Get This Way? Knowledge of the Causes Is Power Over the Disease

➤Flashback➤

Connecting the dots completes a picture of the causes. I had a history of chronic constipation and migraine headaches since childhood. The traditional medical diagnosis was always the same: "stress induced." Through natural health-care, I successfully overcame these debilitating conditions. Symptoms of constipation did not reappear until injuries resulting from a life-threatening fall necessitated taking prescription drugs. As a result of the accident, I was hospitalized and placed in intensive care. I developed blood clots, pulmonary embolism, and was administered oral and I.V. therapy to thin my blood. During my stay in the intensive care unit, I was prescribed drugs for pain, anti-inflammatory drugs and muscle relaxant drugs.

When I entered the hospital I had no muscle pain or fatigue and enjoyed a high level of energy and stamina. I had a successful practice, including occupational and preventive

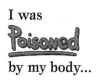
health-care, and enjoyed good quality of life. Shortly after my release from the hospital, I developed what was diagnosed as chronic fatigue. The doctors attributed my symptoms to trauma recuperation. Then my vicious cycle began.

As my complaints grew in intensity, so did the list of prescribed drugs for symptom-care. I was prescribed antidepressant drugs, because I was apparently too impatient to regain my energy and stamina, anti-inflammatory drugs because of muscle pain and decreasing pain tolerance, and muscle relaxing drugs because of my inability to sleep.

Next came the diagnosis of fibromyalgia with the accompanying chronic insomnia. I was told that because I was "under excessive stress" I subsequently developed fibromyalgia. You bet I was under stress! I had very little quality of life. I could only work four hours a day instead of the usual twelve. I was sleep-deprived and my body was so sore it felt like the nerve endings were on top of my skin. How can the pain and frustration be explained to the observer when everything external looks normal?

This drama continued until I determined no one was getting to the causes. We were merely causing more and more drug side effects.

I finally regained a better quality of life through alternative therapies with only minor residues of my past symptoms. I proceeded to complete a Ph.D. in Natural Health and presented my thesis,

What Function Does the Gut Perform?

The function of the gastrointestinal tract, or gut, is complex. Basically, the gut:

- Digests foods.
- Carries nutrients (like vitamins and minerals) attached to carrier proteins across the gut lining into the bloodstream.
- Functions as a major component of the body's detoxification system.
- Contains immunoglobulins (antibodies) that act as the first line of defense against infection.

If the gut is not healthy, neither is the rest of the body.

The gut performs the job of a human chemical factory. It contains billions of intestinal bacteria that have an important effect on human physiology. They produce toxins and antitoxins that alter the chemical composition of foods and drugs. The number of bacteria in the large intestine (colon) is estimated to be a hundred billion. This number exceeds the total number of cells in the human body. Intestinal bacteria perform vital functions by keeping the digestion and assimilation of consumed substances in balance. In LGS, the intestinal lining allows substances and bacteria to leak through into the circulatory system, triggering the body's allergic responses.

Leaky gut is caused by inflammation of the intestinal lining, usually characterized by damage to individual cells. The damaged cells are less able to produce the enzymes and other healthy secretions necessary for effective digestion and absorption of nutrients.

The intestine contains some of the most toxic organisms imaginable (bacteria, fungus, yeast overgrowth, toxic residue from chemicals, bile salts, and parasites). These organisms are responsible for the breakdown of the immune system. A healthy functioning intestine keeps these substances normalized, (in balance), and prevents them from leaking into the bloodstream.

When there is leakage of "bad" bacteria, they enter and surround the connective tissue, creating inflammatory responses. As a result of this inflammation and cell damage, the white blood cells (our Pac-man scavengers of abnormal bacteria) must deal with excessive antigen overload, preventing the cells from doing an effective cleanup.

Destruction of Health
Begins in the Colon

Allow me to take you on a trip through the gastrointestinal tract, or food canal, of the human body.

Ignoring technical anatomical details, the food canal is a muscular tube about ten times the length of the body, measured from the top of the head to the end of the spinal column. The circular muscles of the lips control the upper end of the canal, which is evident when whistling. The mouth and teeth prepare food to undergo the various processes performed in deeper parts. Circular muscles at other points along the canal regulate movements of foodstuffs during the process of digestion. The chief part, the small intestine, is coiled up in the lower cavity of the trunk below the diaphragm. At the lower end of the canal is the colon, wonderfully designed to receive and discharge unused remnants of food and other waste materials from the body. The colon is sacculated, meaning it is formed from a series of connected pouches, unlike the small intestine with its smooth tube of uniform size. At the extreme lower end of the canal is the anus, controlled by circular muscles that act both voluntarily and involuntarily. Both in health and disease these "food gates" have an important relation to digestion and elimination. Respected medical authorities have understood the importance of colon health since the late 19th century.

In this century, the vital role of colon health was generally ignored. Practitioners of alternative medicine and some nutritionally aware physicians are again discussing it as a vital part of the disease process. Modern studies of this part of the intestine show that, by neglect, this temporary reservoir of wastes becomes a veritable breeding place of disease and disorders, many described as "incurable." Professor Keith, an eminent English anatomist, attributes the diseases of the colon to the adoption of a diet unsuited to human anatomy.

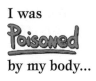
Therefore, we are not only what we eat, but also how we digest and eliminate it.

The colon forms a receptacle for wastes and excretory substances, together with unusable or undigested residues of food and drugs. The collection of waste materials is only an incidental function of the colon. Its important function is to conduct these unusable materials out of the body as fecal wastes.

Constipation

There can be many causes of constipation; however, for the purposes of this book, I'll discuss those related to LGS and the consequences of prescription drug therapies.

Did you know that Americans spend $750,000,000 a year on laxatives? Physicians write more than 1,200,000 prescriptions for constipation complexes annually. Nearly every man, woman, and child living today in a westernized society is constipated. A misconception exists that if you eliminate once a day, you are normal and healthy. Consider this: if you eat three meals a day, and eliminate once (or less) daily, where is the rest of the waste material? Often, the whole length of the colon is completely packed with old hardened fecal matter, leaving a narrow channel that enables only small, soft feces to pass through. This condition is commonly referred to as "tunnel elimination." In other words, fecal matter accumulates on the walls of the colon and eventually attaches, causing the canal of elimination to narrow. Yes, even people with chronic diarrhea have a form of constipation.

To better understand the meaning of the word "constipate," look at its origin. The Latin root is *constipare,* meaning to press together or compact. Therefore, constipation is a condition in which the feces are packed or pressed together. There are three types of constipation.

Common Constipation

This condition exists when the feces passing from the body are overly dry and packed together and elimination of the bowel content is incomplete. Eliminations can be two or more times daily with no additional symptoms. This condition usually results from lack of dietary fiber, irregular eating schedules, lack of moisture, and neglecting the urge to eliminate. Typical American diets consist of less than 12 grams of fiber. Recommendations of fiber intake for proper colon health are 20–35 grams daily. Without proper amounts of fiber, the colon is unable to brush the fecal material from the colon walls. This condition can generally be corrected by increasing dietary fiber, taking the time for regular eliminations, and increasing water consumption. Water is vital in providing sufficient hydration to facilitate elimination.

Concealed Constipation

This type of constipation typically occurs in people suffering from chronic disease. Concealed constipation takes years to develop and most people are not aware of its presence because the bowels move regularly once a day. Symptoms of this kind of constipation include unexplained fatigue, headaches, bad breath, appendicitis, colitis, PMS, anxiety, and depression. The long-term effects are not recognized until secondary symptoms or diseases are diagnosed. More often than not, this constipation is accelerated by lack of exercise, commonly brought on by pain and discomfort from chronic disease or disorders like fibromyalgia, chronic fatigue, and arthritis.

Drug-Induced Constipation

Drug-induced constipation is a potentially serious type of constipation. Symptoms generally manifest within a few days of taking the medication. Drug-induced constipation, in combination with concealed constipation, is a sure prescription for leaky gut. This constipation occurs especially with high-potency painkillers, antacids with aluminum, iron supplements, some narcotics, and antidepressants.

The following are examples of commonly prescribed drugs for inflammation, pain, insomnia, and anxiety, with constipating side effects:

- Hydrocodone/APAP
- Acetaminophen with codeine Naproxen
- Prednisone
- Alprazolam
- Lorazepam
- Amitriptyline
- Trazodone

Laxatives: Short-Term Solution, Long-Range Impact

Laxatives are employed to give immediate bowel relief. Laxatives merely stimulate the bowels to move. Chronic use causes the bowels to become lazy and the muscles become dependent on laxatives to constrict. Taking laxatives is *not* a substitute for fiber in your food. Most laxatives irritate the colon, cause damage to colon walls and nerve cells, and cause the bowels to expel the laxative and anything else loose enough to flow. This action generally makes no specific attempt to expel anything older than the laxative itself. It does *not* dislodge stagnant material within the colon. For this reason, laxatives are a quick fix and have no colon-cleansing benefits. Once the laxative passes through the colon, you're right back where you started (with a plugged-up sewer system), only now you may have the added irritation of the laxative.

If you use laxatives for a prolonged period of time, you'll need to re-train your body to eliminate without the laxative "crutch." Don't ignore your body's urge to defecate, take the time. Proper elimination is imperative to good health. The longer the waste stays in the body, the more toxic material is available to enter the bloodstream.

Helpful Drugs: Serious Side Effects

Non-steroidal Anti-inflammatory Drugs (NSAIDs)

NSAIDs are non-steroidal drugs, as distinguished from those that contain corticosteroids. They are a group of drugs most frequently used to reduce swelling, inflammation, pain, and fever. The drugs work by inhibiting the enzyme cyclooxygenase. This enzyme is responsible for the production of prostaglandins, hormone-like substances involved in the development of pain and inflammation.

In the U.S. alone, 75 million prescriptions for NSAIDs are written annually. Every year an estimated 7,600 people die from the effects, including gastrointestinal bleeding and perforation; that's one death for every 9,210 prescriptions. Another 76,000 are hospitalized; that's one hospitalization for every 921 prescriptions. It is estimated that the resulting effects of gastrointestinal ulcers alone cost $100 million a year. *Medical Advertising News* estimated that 20,000 deaths each year are attributed to NSAID-induced complications, and the number is rapidly growing. According to the medical journal *Lancet*, chronic use of NSAIDs, especially in high doses, increases the permeability or leaking of the colon. This leaking actually creates allergies and contributes to arthritic and inflammatory symptoms, the very reason most people take an NSAID in the first place. This category of drugs comes in many forms, some prescription and many over-the-counter formulations.

The most commonly used NSAIDs are listed below.

- Actron
- Advil
- Aleve
- Aspirin
- ASA
- Ibuprofen

- Indomethacin
- Ketroprofen
- Motrin
- Naprosine
- Naproxen
- Teleprin

RxLists of Indications and Side Effects reports the following common side effects associated with use of NSAIDs:

- Abdominal pain
- Agranulocytosis
- Amblyopia
- Anemia
- Angioedema
- Anorexia
- Aplastic anemia
- Azotemia
- Bleeding
- Blurred vision
- Bronchospasm
- Bullous rash
- Cholestasis
- Constipation
- Corneal deposits
- Diarrhea
- Dizziness
- Drowsiness
- Dyspepsia
- Dyspnea

- Edema
- Elevated hepatic enzymes
- Erythema nodosum
- Exfoliative dermatitis
- Flatulence
- Gastritis
- GI bleeding
- GI perforation
- Granulocytopenia
- Headache
- Hearing loss
- Heart failure
- Hematuria
- Hemolysis
- Hepatic failure
- Hepatitis
- Hyperkalemia
- Hypertension
- Hyperuricemia
- Infection

- Insomnia
- Interstitial nephritis
- Intraventricular disorder
- Hemorrhage
- Jaundice
- Keratitis
- Lethargy
- Leukopenia
- Maculopapular rash
- Malaise
- Melena
- Musculoskeletal inflammation
- Nausea/vomiting
- Nephrotic syndrome
- Occult GI bleeding
- Ocular irritation
- Osteoarthritis
- Palpitations
- Pancreatitis
- Pancytopenia
- Peptic ulcer
- Peripheral edema
- Photosensitivity
- Platelet dysfunction
- Proteinuria
- Pruritus
- Pseudoporphyria
- Purpura
- Renal papillary necrosis
- Retinal hemorrhage
- Reye's syndrome
- Rheumatoid arthritis
- Seizures
- Tachycardia
- Stevens-Johnson syndrome
- Tendonitis
- Thrombocytopenia
- Tinnitus
- Toxic epidermal necrolysis
- Urticaria
- Vasculitis
- Vertigo
- Visual impairment

Steroidal Drugs

Prescription corticosteroids, including prednisone, are commonly used for inflammatory disorders. They are available only by prescription. Use of steroid drugs increases yeast in the digestive tract and is damaging to the liver.

Acetaminophen (Tylenol®)

Acetaminophen products, like Tylenol®, aren't a classic NSAID; however, more than other classes of pain-relief medications, they do have some of the same effects and appear to be closely related to NSAIDs. However, Tylenol® does not specifically appear to affect prostaglandins. Keep in mind that extended use or large doses of acetaminophen may lead to liver damage and, with leaky gut, as with most digestive disorders, the liver function is already compromised.

Over-the-Counter (OTC) Pain Relievers

Stronger NSAIDs require a prescription, but lower-dose NSAIDs, such as formulations containing ibuprofen, are available as OTC preparations and are often thought to be relatively safe by consumers. How many times have you, or someone you know, taken an ibuprofen to relieve the pain of stiffness and swelling? You take these pills regularly, perhaps even daily, without much thought of the impending consequences. After all, "They're available without my doctor's prescription, so they can't be too harmful." Anti-inflammatory drugs such as aspirin, ibuprofen, and many over-the-counter drugs are *not harmless.* They're drugs!

Dozens of OTC pain medications may initially appear to be much less likely to upset the stomach lining than stronger prescription drugs, but these medications are just as damaging to the intestinal lining. They are still NSAIDs and cause damage to the lining by blocking the prostaglandins stimulating tissue repair. *Keep in mind that while NSAIDs act as anti-inflammatories in the bloodstream and body tissues, they have an irritant or caustic effect in the gastrointestinal tract and damage the lining of the microvilli in the intestinal wall. NSAIDs are a direct cause of leaky gut syndrome and can lead to food and environmental sensitivities and inflammatory disorders.* Consumers may not recognize that damage or irritation to the colon and digestive systems has occurred. They are overwhelmed dealing with the symptoms of pain and inflammation and concerned with immediate relief. If side effects of NSAIDs are suspected, consumers commonly look for the most common, quick, old-fashioned solution—aspirin.

Aspirin

It is common in today's society to take a couple of aspirin for a headache, to calm down your pain of arthritis or fibromyalgia, or to get rid of all those body aches after a day of gardening, shopping or driving. The Aspirin Foundation boasts that this chemical "has probably been taken, at one time or another, by almost every human being on earth." Americans gulp down an estimated 30 million aspirin tablets a day.

Americans are not alone in their overindulgence of aspirin. While in Europe, I was amazed to see the quantities being consumed: in Britain as a powdered form, in France as rectal suppositories, and in Spain as an effervescent.

Chemical companies produce over 100 million aspirin tablets a year. Consumers are bombarded with commercial and professional advice to consume "an aspirin a day" to prevent heart attacks. The Physician's Health Study reported that the preventive aspect of aspirin used for clinical studies was a buffered form containing magnesium as in Bufferin™. Research reported that the magnesium component, not the aspirin, is the specific protector of the heart. Magnesium is necessary for every cell in the body. It dilates blood vessels, aids the absorption of potassium into the cells (preventing irregularities of heartbeat), and may assist in keeping the blood cells from sticking together (thrombosis). Autopsies of the heart muscle following death by heart attack almost always reveal that the heart muscle is deficient in magnesium.

A British study using *plain aspirin* revealed aspirin may lower the incidence of heart attack by the anticoagulant (blood thinning) effect. However, it was not reported that every time you take aspirin you bleed a little into the gut. A microscope will show the bowel movement of someone on daily aspirin has blood in it every time. If it's happening in your intestinal tract, how do you know it's not happening in your brain? Doesn't it make you wonder what else might be precipitated by chronic aspirin intake? Or, how many fatal hemorrhages of the brain, spleen, liver, intestine, or lung occur after an accident, because the blood has been thinned by excessive aspirin consumption? Many of my clients, as well as myself, are being advised by their physicians to take daily doses of aspirin, especially after an accident like mine resulting in thrombosis. Many of my senior clients are advised to take aspirin daily as a preventive measure against diseases associated with aging.

It is alarming to sit on my side of the health-care desk and listen to the long list of symptoms that are associated with regular aspirin consumption. When clients make the decision to stop the daily aspirin routine, many of the symptoms disappear. For example, during a routine health assessment consultation, a client will describe occasional rectal bleeding. They reported it to their physician during routine check-ups. The medical rectal exams show no evident cause (polyps, hemorrhoids, etc.). When I ask about aspirin consumption, most answer, "Yes, daily, I've been told it's good for me." When clients decide to stop the aspirin for a trial period, they report that no rectal bleeding occurred during the test period. When they resume daily intake of aspirin, rectal bleeding is again evident. This tells me a lot, and it should send up red flags for you, too.

What is even more alarming are findings published in the *British Medical Journal.* The journal reported the conclusions of California researchers: in older men and women who take aspirin every day the chances of developing ischemic heart disease double. Ischemic heart disease accounts for a wide range of symptoms caused by blockage of cardiac arteries. The study also found that aspirin users were more likely to develop kidney and colon cancer. These studies, as well as personal and professional experience, make me question how many other disorders might have started from the use of aspirin? Maybe for many of us aspirin began the "gut reaction" of intestinal disorders. It's a thought worth digesting.

Prescription Pain Medication

We take pain medications to treat the inflammation and pain, which, in turn, causes damage to the intestinal lining, leading to more inflammation and pain. The pain may temporarily be reduced with the use of pain medication, but the effects of the damage are yet to present themselves as a manifested disease or disorder. Also, there is often tissue or organ damage caused by the chemical toxins, setting up a perfect environment for subsequent *Candida* yeast overgrowth. After taking drugs for a prolonged period of time, laboratory testing is essential to determine the existence and degree of *Candida* yeast overgrowth. These tests are readily available through health-care practitioners (see Chapter 6 for resources).

As if the described toxic effects aren't enough, constipation is also a side effect of many pain medications, especially codeine-containing drugs such as hydrocodone/APAP.

Stress and Your Digestive System

Stresses do not directly cause LGS or associated digestive disorders. However, they contribute to development of the disorders when the body's resistance is lowered.

Dr. Hans Selye refers to inflammatory disease as one of the "stress diseases." Adrenal exhaustion from prolonged stress is one of the major causes leading to the development of inflammatory and digestive disorders. The pituitary and/or adrenal glands, due to prolonged stress and consequent impaired metabolism, are no longer able to function normally and produce cortisone, desoxycortisone, aldosterone, and other natural hormones. Severe hormonal imbalance will be the result, leading to further metabolic derangement and severely lowered resistance to stress from infections, drugs, toxic substances in foods, etc. As famed nutritionist Adele Davis said, "Meeting the demands of stress" should be your first consideration. The best way to accomplish this is to adopt a self-care life-style by eating a diet rich in organic unprocessed fresh vegetables, fruits, grain, and seeds.

Stress plays a major role in digestive disorders. Continued stress in our mind, body, and spirit affects the body's ability to heal. One of the body's reactions to stress is to slow down digestion and reduce blood flow to the digestive organs, straining the ability of the gastrointestinal tract to function at full capacity.

Candida
(Systemic Yeast Overgrowth)
and Dysbiosis

*How Did I
Get This
Way?
Knowledge
of the Causes
Is Power
Over the
Disease*

85

Your Internal Ecosystem

Just as the forest must have enough vegetation to filter out the toxins in our environment, so our body needs to contain an abundance of friendly bacteria to balance the unfriendly bacteria. Nowadays, our intestinal ecosystems are subjected to sugars, refined foods, antibiotics, corticosteroids, and barrages of drugs that disturb or destroy our intestinal balance.

What is Dysbiosis?

Dysbiosis was named by Dr. Eli Metchnikoff in the early 1900s. He won the Nobel Prize in 1908 for his work on *lactobacilli* (good bacteria) and their role in immunity. He was a colleague of Louis Pasteur and succeeded him as the director of the Pasteur Institute in Paris. The origin of the term "dysbiosis" came from the word "symbiosis," which means to live together in mutual harmony. Dysbiosis was derived from the original term by the prefix "dys," meaning *not*. Thus, dysbiosis is an unbalanced intestinal tract. Beneficial bacteria combat the overgrowth of yeast, fungi, parasites, and health-depleting bacteria.

Candidiasis (Candida)

The most common form of dysbiosis is *Candida,* a fungal infection. *Candida* is a normally occurring fungus living in the mucous membranes, especially in the digestive tract and vagina. It is also found in the sinuses, ear canals, and genitourinary tract. The healthy body can handle normal amounts of this fungus, but large amounts contribute to the decline of digestive health. In healthy conditions, the *Candida* yeasts live in harmony with the other organisms in the intestinal tract. Anything that weakens the immune system encourages the growth of *Candida.* When this yeast outnumbers the other bacteria (*Candida albicans* overgrowth), the condition is called "candidiasis."

Causes of Candida

There are multiple causes allowing this yeast to grow out of control. Our western civilization is accustomed to a diet of fast and convenient foods, rich in sugar, yeast, and preservatives. The extensive use of antibiotics also results in yeast overgrowth. Antibiotics destroy both friendly and disease-causing bacteria. Yeast is *not* killed by antibiotics, but flourishes in the resulting *imbalance* of intestinal bacteria. After antibiotic therapy is complete, the reduced population of friendly bacteria allows yeast to multiply at alarming rates, releasing excessive toxins into the body. *Candida* overgrowth, in turn, releases toxins that weaken the body's immune system. In the case of LGS, digestive and immune disorders, the already weakened immune system now has the added toxins leaking through the intestinal wall.

Symptoms Associated with Candida:

- Extreme fatigue
- Lethargy
- Foggy thinking
- Depression
- Yeast infections
- Poor memory
- Mood swings
- Muscle weakness
- Allergies
- Athlete's foot
- Nail fungus
- Bloating and gas
- Nasal congestion
- Post-nasal drip
- Vinegar cravings
- Skin fungus infections
- Jock itch
- Carbohydrate cravings
- Sugar cravings
- Unexplained anxiety
- Low blood sugar

- Symptoms worse in damp, muggy, moldy places
- Sensitivities to cigarette, perfume, fabric odors
- Generalized environmental sensitivities
- Recurring sinus and ear infections

Few health-care providers are aware that many of today's disorders are yesterday's yeast. Leaky gut is the breakdown of the gut lining, allowing toxins to leak through, and *Candida* thrives in a toxic environment. It's been my experience that you don't see a person with leaky gut without systemic yeast overgrowth, and most people with excessive yeast overgrowth have leaky gut to some degree.

Parasitic Involvement: What's Bugging You?

Yes, I know this will open a "can of worms," but parasites and abnormal bacteria irritate the intestinal lining, and therefore are willing contributors to intestinal disorders. Parasites are opportunistic invaders. When our intestinal and immune system is in healthy balance, there is less opportunity for parasitic infestation. Antibiotics kill bacteria indiscriminately, both the good and the disease-causing bacteria, disrupting the intestinal ecosystem. Our immune system is our first line of defense against invading bacteria, viruses, and parasites. Patients with compromised immune systems are at greater risk for opportunistic infections.

Parasites and worms are scavenger organisms living within, upon, or at the expense of a host organism, without contributing to the survival of the host. They reside in the gastrointestinal tract and feed on toxins and waste material in the body. The most common are roundworms (hookworms, pinworms, and threadworms) and tapeworms. The danger of these uninvited visitors is the waste materials expelled into the host body that are extremely toxic and even deadly. Parasites and worms may be associated with many diseases. Unfortunately, most medical professionals never check for them. Parasites are generally associated with AIDS, colon disorders, some types of cancer, chronic fatigue syndrome, irritable bowel syndrome, and *Candida*. Frequent use of antibiotics, a diet low in fiber and high in sugar, and some prescription drugs reduce beneficial intestinal flora and provide a nourishing environment for parasites and worms to flourish. If you have a chronic digestive condition that resists treatment and onset of symptoms occurred after a trip to South America, Asia, Africa, China, or tropical islands, you very likely have parasitic involvement.

One common type of infection, *giardiasis*, is so common in some areas that the entire population hosts this microorganism. Also known as "Montezuma's Revenge" or "Delhi Belly," this condition causes violent cramping and diarrhea that continues despite the use of over-the-counter medications. *Giardia* organisms are regularly found in mountain streams. More alarming is the fact that they infect many of our city water systems, since *Giardia is not killed by chlorination.* Water is the main avenue for spread of *giardiasis* in this country and abroad. For the past several years, the Center for Disease Control (CDC) has reported that the *Giardia* organism is the most prevalent cause of waterborne disease in America. According to the Environmental Protection Agency (EPA), outbreaks in treated municipal water are doubling every five years.

Symptoms of *giardiasis* may last for weeks or months and can linger, masquerading as other disorders, for years. Recent references in scientific literature suggest these parasites may be the primary cause of allergies. This theory is revolutionary and additional research continues to determine just how large a role parasites play in allergies. Parasites cause damage to the lining of the digestive tract, allowing large molecules to enter the bloodstream, hence "leaky gut." This reaction can then provoke an antigenic response.

Many physicians request generalized parasitology testing on random stool samples; however, this type of testing is not very accurate. It's been my experience that the most accurate testing is done by labs specializing in parasitology testing and requires two or more samples.

Innovative options for testing and healing are discussed in Chapters 6 and 7.

6

Identifying the Problem: Uncovering What Traditional Diagnosis Does NOT

Innovative Alternative Testing

The tests listed below are not ordinary tests performed at your local medical laboratory or hospital. However, more and more laboratories are offering these optional tests as demand increases. Your health-care practitioner or nutritionally aware physician will be familiar with these innovative testing methods. These laboratories offer complete information packages and test kits, and offer your physician assistance in interpreting the results.

Live Cell Variable Projection Microscopy

This test pioneered the concept of Oxidology, the study of reactive oxygen toxic species (ROTS) in health and disease as a precise medical subspecialty. Bradford Research Institute has the most advanced variable projection multi-phase optical microscopy system available. This instrument has made possible the correlation of pathology with the dynamics of peripheral blood morphology, yielding unique insights into clinical and subclinical mechanisms.

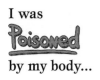
Live cell analysis is a unique and innovative way to obtain a screening perspective of amount and general location of the oxidative processes at work within the body. In addition, it shows hormones, enzymes, and other by-products of biological stresses at work. Diseases demonstrated are often chronic. However, progressive, acute, sub-acute and degenerative conditions are visible as well. This unique analysis has the ability, among other things, to reveal the condition of the immune system. Some of the constituents clearly observed are white blood cells and their activity; extent of foreign antigens and microbes with the serum; and the strength, condition, and movement of red blood cells. These three major components judge the strength of the immune system and might possibly indicate a progressive disease process at work.

A second series of drops is placed on a second slide taken from the same finger prick at the same time, and allowed to dry. This gives further insight into the general location within the body of pathological activity, particular processes, toxin build-up, and length of time it has been present.

This type of analysis acts as an educational "feedback mechanism" for the client. Changes in the makeup of the blood cells, improvement in toxin amounts, etc. may be viewed periodically as a progress indicator.

The analysis serves as a barometer for the client and health-care provider, enabling each to monitor health and the changes taking place.

The tests are performed by clinicians and practitioners worldwide, certified by Bradford Research Institute. The following material is used with permission from Great Smokies Diagnostic Institute. (See explanation of how the test is performed in "My Story.")

Intestinal Permeability Testing

Most of the non-invasive permeability-testing techniques are simple and reliable and can be used to assess many clinical conditions. This test determines underlying problems linked to GI function. It directly measures how well two non-metabolized sugar molecules, mannitol and lactulose, permeate the intestinal mucosa. Low levels of mannitol and lactulose indicate mal-absorption. Elevated levels of lactulose and mannitol are indicative of general increased permeability and leaky gut phenomena. This test requires an overnight fast.

Comprehensive Digestive Stool Analysis (CDSA)

This test evaluates digestion, absorption, intestinal function, and the microbial flora such as *Candida* (yeast overgrowth). The CDSA uncovers the fundamental causes of many acute and chronic symptoms and is used in the evaluation of various gastrointestinal symptoms or systemic illnesses that may have started in the intestines. Because illnesses are often not discernable from symptoms, the CDSA is a valuable means for identifying critical imbalances previously unsuspected.

Comprehensive Parasitology Testing

This test can uncover parasitic infections associated with systemic complaints. The diagnosis of most parasitic infections depends on the laboratory. For intestinal parasites, morphological demonstration of diagnostic stages is the principal means of diagnosis. Computer-enhanced video microscopy aids in identification and provides the physician and patient with an actual picture of organisms found.

Liver Detoxification Profile

This test assesses the body's capacity to carry out detoxification through functional challenges (caffeine, acetaminophen, and salicylate) which evaluate specific aspects of the detoxification process and free radical damage. These functional assessments provide a comprehensive profile of the body's detoxification capacity and potential susceptibility to oxidative damage. It is a good way to assess the effects of pharmaceutical drugs and herbal substances.

Note: All referenced tests must be ordered by a physician or health-care practitioner.

7

Healing the Leaky Gut Naturally: Not Medicine as Usual

Once you've identified the problem with the appropriate recommended testing options, you can start your journey to wellness.

This chapter discusses effective therapies for healing your digestive system. It is advisable to take any supplements under the strict guidance of a qualified health-care professional who can select the most appropriate course of action for your particular situation. Many people attempting self-treatment, or with the advice of well-meaning sales people without qualified training, do not take the correct products or dosages. Under the guidance of a qualified health professional, you should expect to see some improvement within the first thirty days. However, it's been my experience, and that of the thousands of clients I've consulted with, that four to six months is necessary for significant reversing of symptoms and im-

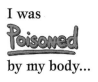
provement in total quality of life. Healing digestive disorders requires a true commitment and life-style change, but considering the options, the majority of my clients and I have chosen the road to recovery via the natural highway.

Strategic Healing

Much has been written about specific categories for healing the leaky gut. The following recommendations represent the approach that allowed me to repair the leaky gut and regain quality of life. It is imperative that you have a health-care practitioner who is knowledgeable and flexible in mapping your road to recovery.

Systemic Cleaning (Detoxifying)

Therapeutic Food

One of the most effective systemic detoxification products, in my clinical experience, is BioInflammatory® by BioGenesis®. It is available through your healthcare provider (see product reference).

BioInflammatory® is a medical food powder designed to support gastro-intestinal healing while removing toxins from your nervous system, connective and fatty tissues. It assists your liver in converting an insoluble toxin, hard to remove, to a soluble toxin, easily removed. It's specialty nutrients are used to enhance chelation and clearing of both metabolic toxins and xenobiotic (environmental) toxins. It is a balanced ratio of protein, carbohydrate and fats to help maintain healthy blood sugar levels and energy. Its base is a hypoallergenic rice protein concentrate free of wheat, rye, oats, barley, corn, dairy, egg and peanut. No artificial colors, fillers or flavors are used.

Skin Brushing

Skin brushing is a highly effective technique for cleansing the lymphatic system. The gastrointestinal cleaning softens hardened mucoid in the lymphatic system, as well as in the intestines. Skin brushing done concurrently with a gastrointestinal cleaning program improves overall detoxification.

The skin is the largest organ of elimination. It plays a major role in ridding your body of the toxins and impurities that are potential sources of illness. It is estimated that the skin eliminates over one pound of waste per day. Isn't that enough to make you want to brush away those toxins? Daily skin brushing is a vital part of an intestinal cleansing program. The skin excretes toxins and poisons present in the body, as do the kidneys and bowels. Dry skin brushing stimulates the sweat glands and increases blood circulation to underlying organs and tissues of the body. Today's sedentary life-style, general lack of exercise, and use of antiperspirants keep people from suffi-ciently perspiring. As a result, toxins and metabolic waste products become trapped in the body in-stead of being released through sweat. Dry skin brushing opens up the pores, allowing your body to breathe and enhance proper organ function.

Types of Skin Brush

The brush used should be a long-handled, bath-type brush. It is essential that it contain only natural vegetable bristles. Synthetic brushes should be com-pletely avoided for this purpose, as they can irritate the skin. You can purchase a quality skin brush through health-food stores and some beauty supply outlets and pharmacies. Keep the brush dry and *never* use it for bathing.

How to Brush Your Skin

The brush must be dry, as well as the body. The best time to brush is before taking a bath or shower. Begin by brushing from the outermost points (your hands and feet) toward the center of your body. Pass the brush once over every part of the body surface except the face. There should be no back and forth motion, circular motion, scrubbing, or massaging; one clean sweep is all that is needed. A slight flushing of the skin is normal due to the increased circulation, but if your skin turns red you are brushing too hard. The total process takes less than two or three minutes. Skin brushing should be performed once or twice per day. It would take thirty minutes or more of lufa or Turkish towel massage to get similar benefits. When you're finished, take a warm bath or shower. You will feel an invigorating, tingling sensation throughout your body.

Illustration of Skin Brushing

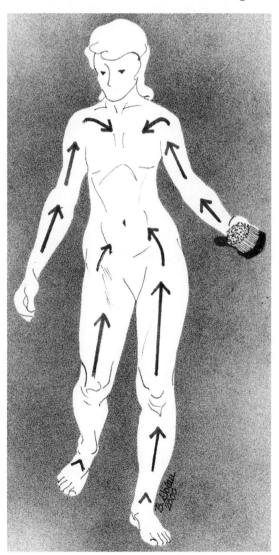

It is common for your stools to contain a large amount of lymph mucoid a day or two after beginning skin brushing. This represents an emptying out of the backlog of fresh lymph mucoid present in the lymphatic system and is a lymph-purifying effect.

Colon Health: "Waste Management"

Colon hydrotherapy saved my life. The detoxifying effects were proven when colon hydrotherapy stopped the frightening symptoms of anaphylactic shock.

Autointoxication is the process by which the body literally poisons itself by maintaining a cesspool of decaying matter in the colon. The toxins released by the decay process get into the bloodstream and travel to all parts of the body. Every cell in the body is affected, and because the toxins weaken the entire system, autointoxication and many forms of "incurable diseases" get their start in the colon. An eminent French physician, Bouchard, coined the word "autointoxication" and described the various ways diseases may be produced by poisons generated in the body. He called special attention to the intestines, especially the colon, as a prolific source of poisons. Still another source of intestinal poisons is the putrefaction of that portion of the protein of food that fails to undergo absorption.

It is entirely possible for a person to suffer from intestinal toxemia without constipation, as in cholera morbus, the diarrheas of infancy, chronic diarrhea, and colitis; but it is impossible to have constipation without intestinal autointoxication. Intestinal poisoning not manifesting immediate visible effects appear in disorders such as fibromyalgia, chronic fatigue, lupus, and arthritis.

There are two effective ways of cleaning the colon: colon hydrotherapy and enemas.

What Is Colon Hydrotherapy?

Colon hydrotherapy is the safe, gentle infusion of water into the colon via the rectum, administered by a certified colon hydrotherapist. The average charge is between $45 and $75 per session. No chemicals or drugs are involved and the entire therapy is both relaxing and effective. During therapy the client lies on a custom treatment table in complete comfort. From the hydrotherapy equipment, a small disposable speculum is gently inserted into the rectum, through which warm filtered water passes into the colon.

Modern state-of-the-art colon hydrotherapy units employ multi-stage water purification systems and individual disposables that eliminate any possible contamination to the client from a previous treatment. A lighted viewing tube allows both the client and therapist to witness the elimination. These are closed systems, so waste is discretely transported into the drain line without offensive odor and without compromising the dignity of the individual. After each therapy session, the unit is thoroughly cleansed and disinfected in preparation for future use.

A skilled colon hydrotherapist will use several fills and releases of water, as well as light massage techniques, to dislodge toxic waste matter adhering to the walls of the colon. The dislodged fecal impactions are then gently washed away through the system's waste disposal hose.

During the therapy, water temperature and pressure will be monitored by the therapist and can be varied to stimulate muscular contraction (peristalsis) in the colon. This is very important to help the sluggish colon.

Properly administered colon hydrotherapy is not addictive but therapeutic; it encourages the restoration of the colon's natural function by strengthening peristalsis.

Each colon hydrotherapy session lasts approximately forty-five minutes and should require at least one hour. Initially, a series of six to twelve separate therapy sessions is normally recommended to begin achieving the maximum cleansing benefits. Depending on the toxicity and level of reactions, colon hydrotherapy sessions need to be custom-tailored by a health-care practitioner. Normally they are administered once a week for several weeks. Most often in acute digestive disorders, as in my case, three therapy sessions a week for several weeks are administered to control anaphylactic shock and acute reactions. This helps eliminate fecal matter lodged in the colon for weeks, months, and in most cases years, and to keep the client properly hydrated. As healing occurs and reactions subside, the therapy sessions are scheduled further and further apart until a maintenance level is accomplished. The optimum maintenance therapy is once every three to four months.

With colon hydrotherapy, the entire large intestine is cleansed and the therapeutic benefits are much greater than those achieved with an enema. Enema cleansing is effective in the rectum area and, due to the body's natural desire to expel, is limited in duration. Over-the-counter suppositories stimulate expulsion of the contents of the rectum but contribute to dehydration, which may exacerbate a constipated condition. During typical colon hydrotherapy sessions, about twenty-five to thirty-five gallons of water are transported into and out of the colon. Using a combination of abdominal massage (if consented), reflexology, breathing instruction, and relaxation techniques, the colon therapist is often able to promote elimination of a great volume of toxic waste not otherwise possible through individual efforts. *Just one colon hydrotherapy session may be equivalent to having twenty or thirty regular bowel movements.* Eliminations during subsequent therapy sessions can be even more substantial as older, hardened, impacted feces are dislodged from the colon walls.

The colon hydrotherapist will carefully evaluate the client's progress during each session and will coordinate therapies with health-care professionals.

At the onset of therapy, clients with chronic conditions may experience some fatigue. Over an

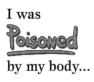
extended period of time, most people feel a heightened energy and vitality, with the subsequent reduction or elimination of the related generalized pain, inflammation, and abdominal discomfort.

Colon hydrotherapy provides a proven way to cleanse the colon, thereby increasing the healing process and maintaining optimal health. Remember that maintaining good health is an ongoing process requiring diligence. Your general health probably declined over a period of time; don't expect an immediate return to health. What you *can* expect is a steady improvement and reduction of symptoms.

Colon hydrotherapy can be most beneficial for restoring good health by:

- Clearing the colon of old, hardened waste material and harmful toxins.
- Restoring proper pH balance to the body.
- Stimulating the immune system.
- Allowing freer passage of nutrients into the blood.
- Increasing prevention of toxic absorption via healthy mucosa.
- Providing a favorable environment for bacteria and micro-flora for digestion.
- Strengthening peristaltic activity in the colon and rectum.
- Promoting a return of normal, regular bowel movements.

Millions of people in this country who suffer a myriad of health problems may never even consider the source of their problems as a toxic, sluggish colon. This is not surprising. The traditional treatment of health disorders, disease symptoms, and disease management using pharmaceuticals and surgery may completely obscure the root cause of recurring health problems.

Enemas

The invention of this instrument, so essential in maintaining health, belongs to an Italian, Gatenaria, whose name ought to find a modest place together with his countrymen Columbus, Galileo, Gioja, and other eminent and illustrious Italians. Gatenaria was a professor at Pavia, where he died in 1496 after spending several years perfecting his instrument. *The British Medical Journal,* in the late 1800s, describes the invention of the enema apparatus as an epoch in pharmacy as important as the discovery of America in the history of human civilization.

Prior to World War II, it was typical for physicians to recommend enemas for preventive and therapeutic value. Before the drug boom took over in the 1920s, enemas continued to be widely written about internationally. In fact, coffee enemas were in the guidebook of medicine, *The Merck Manual of Medical Information,* until 1977. Coffee enemas were used for generations as a way to purge the colon, liver, and gallbladder. (With leaky gut, the stimulation of coffee can trigger a reaction. I recommend plain, purified water.) Enema therapy was removed from *The Merck Manual of Medical Information* merely because the space was needed to list all the new drugs on the market. Drugs have a higher profit margin than an enema kit!

Whether enemas are the preferred method of colon irrigation, or an adjunct to professional colon hydrotherapy, colon cleansing has a beneficial effect on most ailments, sickness, or disease. The ancient "natural hygiene" philosophy widely discussed in historical medical books is that all disease is merely a question of *toxicity*. Today's reluctance to use enema therapy stems from a lack of knowledge of its function and purpose. Our "quick fix" attitudes and demand for symptom-care, rather than health care, help fuel this reluctance.

You can purchase a reusable enema kit in most drug stores. If you choose to use a disposable hospital bag, you can purchase one at a medical supply store; however, you'll still need the tube and assembly unit. Be sure the water is boiled or distilled. The bag should *not be over eighteen inches higher than the body,* as the enema solution can run into the colon too fast and cause cramping or bloating. Lubricate the tube with pure Vitamin E. Some lubricant jellies have ingredients that may cause an irritation or reaction. The colon hydrotherapist or health-care practitioner can help with specifics on positioning and self-massage techniques to assist in therapy.

Natural Bulking Agent for Colon Cleansing

Everywhere you look, from magazines and newspapers to radio and television, fiber and fiber products are widely talked about and highly advertised. We are literally being bombarded with commercials and advertisements telling us that eating more fiber is not only the right thing to do, but will solve practically all of life's problems. Fiber is essential; however, all fiber and fiber containing complexes are *not* created equal. Know the facts and *not* just the "sales pitch."

Fiber supplements should *not* be used on a regular basis as a substitute for an appropriate diet. The colon cleansing and fiber-bulking products described in this chapter are used for therapeutic purposes and should be monitored by a health-care practitioner.

►Flashback◄

I tried dozens of fiber agents and reacted to most of them. Not only did some ingredients precipitate a reaction, they failed to produce regular, sufficient eliminations.

The product best tolerated with the highest degree of benefit for my clients and myself is Coloklysis™ Colon Cleanse, manufactured by PhysioLogics® Laboratory (see product reference list). *The results obtained with this product are astounding!* It produces extraordinary results in removing old, putrefied colonic matter. I haven't found another product that comes close to the results achieved with Coloklysis™ Colon Cleanse.

➤Flashback➤

To further prove the effectiveness of this colon cleanse, I went so far as to have a medical laboratory perform a pathologic microscopic examination of eliminated rectal tissue. I passed the examined specimen after only two weeks on Coloklysis™ Colon Cleanse. My suspicions were correct: "old necrotic tissue," which can be likened to a gangrenous condition. With leaky gut, not only was there excessive toxic waste in my colon, it was now circulating throughout my body. My body was poisoning itself! There's no way of knowing how long this matter sat in my colon becoming more and more toxic. What I do know is that thanks to Colokylsis™ Colon Cleanse, the gangrenous mass detached and was eliminated. No other product I used had been able to achieve that result.

During a colon cleanse, I always recommend my clients examine their elimination to see how much the colon has packed away and putrefied. This decaying waste material affects other vital organ systems, especially the kidneys and liver, because of circulating toxicity and their overwork trying to deal with the poisons. As we glance at our bowel movements, we see the brown color of fecal matter and assume that's all it is. During an effective cleansing program, what you see on the outside is not necessarily what it is. Don't judge elimination by its cover.

At first, the idea of examining your stools may be difficult to accept. However, the majority of my clients report that after having participated in such an exercise, which takes less than a minute, the results are so apparent (seeing is believing) they actually look forward to watching the progress of ridding their bodies of the accumulated poisonous toxic waste. We've all had to add some humor to this process, so we coined the phrase "chop sewage."

I started out attempting to find a discrete method of examining my bowel movements. I found that using a pair of chopsticks worked very well because it allowed me to break apart the fecal matter in the commode bowl to examine what was being eliminated. I keep the cleaned chopsticks in a small can or receptacle behind the commode and use them each time I eliminate. Chopsticks made of wood are usually disposable but, for this purpose, can be reused several days if thoroughly rinsed—another contribution to recycling! They provide an invaluable examination tool. Plastic chop sticks are also available and easier to clean. I finally located the ultimate chop sticks for this purpose, made of stainless steel.

While examining your elimination, you may see anything from very large chunks of stringy, black, fibrous mucous, covered with parasites, to putrefied slabs of matter that look like raw beefsteak.

Healing the
Leaky Gut
Naturally:
Not Medicine
as Usual

109

Coloklysis™ Colon Cleanse acts as the scouring pad to loosen all the decayed toxic waste attached to the intestinal walls. With leaky gut you have additional toxins circulating; consequently, the more accumulated waste removed, the sooner you'll be on the road to recovery.

I recommend examining your eliminations ("chop sewage" method) one week before starting the Coloklysis™ Colon Cleanse. This gives you a good comparison of your eliminations before and after the cleansing program. Once you get over the initial idea of examining your stools, you'll be motivated by seeing the progress of your body eliminating substances that are poisoning you and preventing you from achieving optimum health.

For this gastrointestinal cleansing program to stay effective for periodic use throughout your life, you should not perform it more than necessary to keep the alimentary tract cleaned. It should *always be used and monitored by a health-care professional.* An initial period of three months is generally recommended; however, that period can be extended depending upon your specific situation and the advice of your health-care practitioner. Once the cleanse is completed, you can perform the program every six to twelve months for the minimum time needed to remove the recent accumulations (usually one month twice annually). The dosage will vary depending on condition and tolerance. *Do not* attempt to use a product like Coloklysis™ Colon Cleanse without professional monitoring.

Healthy vs. Unhealthy Stool

It is easy to identify a healthy stool. Generally, a medium-brown, well-formed, floating stool with no odor signifies the presence of a healthy, slightly acidic colon pH and the predominance of friendly lactobacteria-type intestinal flora. A sinking, dark-colored stool with a bad or foul odor guarantees overgrowth of unfriendly intestinal flora and an alkaline colon.

Many people assume it is normal for the stool to have a bad odor. On the contrary, a malodorous stool is perhaps the most significant factor indicating a putrefactive colon flora. The stool will naturally vary from day to day, depending on diet and other factors. However, you should expect a consistent pattern indicating a healthy stool with slight color variations but no dramatic changes or odor.

Daily Fiber Bulking Agents

There are a number of good bulking agents that can be taken on a daily basis for months at a time. I like the bulking effects of Coloklysis Daily™, also by PhysioLogics®. It provides a gentle, yet very effective, support in colon detoxification without the deep action of a colon cleanse. Equally important as fiber, it contains ingredients to support healing, like fructooligosaccharides (FOS), aloe vera, ginger, and l-glutamine.

Several good fiber bulking products contain bentonite clay with the fiber bulking ingredients. These combinations are valuable because of the ability of

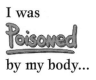
bentonite clay to absorb many times its own weight and volume in toxic material to be eliminated in the feces. However, for leaky gut, products containing bentonite clay should be introduced slowly and for short periods of time. It's been my experience that too much bentonite clay can cause constipation, defeating the original purpose for which it was taken.

Main Functions of Dietary Fiber:

- Improves bowel function by absorbing water in the intestines to provide bulk and soften stools, thereby preventing straining.
- Absorbs and eliminates toxins and prevents constipation, hemorrhoids, and diverticulitis.
- Reduces transit time (see explanation in the following section "Bowel Transit Time").
- Lowers cholesterol. Oat bran fiber, psyllium, and guar gum can lower the harmful low density lipids (LDL) and raise the valuable protective high density lipids (HDL) cholesterol.
- Reduces the risk of colon and rectal cancer. This is generally recognized by the American Cancer Society and the Surgeon General of the United States.
- Improves diabetes. Fiber slows the digestion of fats. It is believed that fiber reduces the amount of insulin needed.

- Acts as an appetite suppressant and reduces the absorption of fats. It draws water into the intestinal system, creating the sensation of fullness with less caloric intake, thus aiding weight loss.

Bowel Transit Time

Ideally, food should take ten to twelve hours to pass into the colon. Most western (low in fiber) diets have an average transit time of sixty-five to one hundred hours (three to ten days, or nine to thirty-six meals). This undigested backed-up body waste is absorbed into the bloodstream and causes autointoxication. Just imagine the volume of thirty-six digested meals composting in your digestive system! The volume of that much waste material could fill a three to five gallon container. Remember, if you're consuming three meals a day, and only eliminating once, the remainder is becoming toxic waste, and your body is the housing for it. Is it any wonder we're so toxic?

Supporting Your Lymphatic System

Without our lymphatic system, we could not live; yet most people barely hear about it or understand its complex work.

The lymph system is closely related to the cardiovascular system, although its major function in the body is as a defense mechanism. It filters out disease-causing organisms, manufactures white blood cells, and generates antibodies. It is a system important in the distribution of fluid and nutrients all over the body because it drains off excess fluids and protein, left behind by capillary circulation, to prevent tissues from swelling.

The fluid that circulates in the system is called lymph. Derived from blood plasma, but clearer and more watery, lymph seeps through the capillary walls to fill tissue spaces. Besides lymph, the system includes lymphatic capillaries, larger vessels, lymph nodes, glands, spleen, tonsils, and thymus.

Lymph vessels are located throughout the body and are more numerous than blood vessels. Lymph is the inner excretory mechanism of the body. The lymphatic system, four times larger than the blood system, provides the means for each individual cell in the body to get rid of waste. Lymphatic capillaries are vessels that are scattered throughout the body. Their job is to collect surplus fluid and transport it to two terminal vessel stations. The first, the thoracic duct, is the lymphatic system's main duct, which lies along the spine and enters a large vein on the left, close to the heart. The second, the right lymphatic duct, enters a subclavian vein on the right side.

Substances resulting from cellular metabolism are extruded from the cell and removed through the lymph; however, lymph handles only cell wastes. When the blood is also dumping waste toxins from the intestinal tract into the lymph system via the liver, the lymph becomes overworked and its filtering/neutralizing function is decreased.

Lymph and lymphatic vessels come into much more intimate relationships with metabolic tissues than the blood. However, unlike the blood system that uses the heart as a pump, the lymph system, like veins, relies on skeletal muscle contractions to pump the lymph along.

Illustration of Entire Lymphatic System

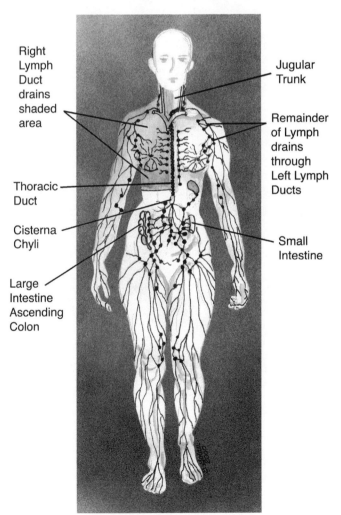

Right Lymph Duct drains shaded area

Jugular Trunk

Remainder of Lymph drains through Left Lymph Ducts

Thoracic Duct

Cisterna Chyli

Small Intestine

Large Intestine Ascending Colon

Hepatic Portal System

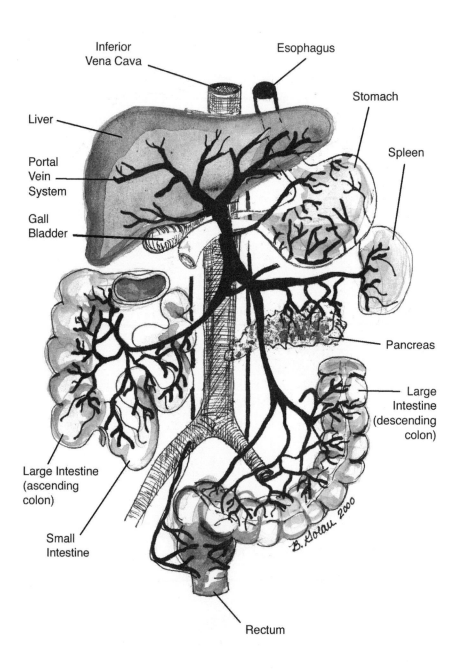

Inferior Vena Cava

Esophagus

Stomach

Spleen

Liver

Portal Vein System

Gall Bladder

Pancreas

Large Intestine (descending colon)

Large Intestine (ascending colon)

Small Intestine

Rectum

B. Jolau 2000

Massage and Lymphatic Stimulation

A toxic bowel leaks poisons through smaller veins that gradually join together until they form one large vein called the portal vein, which goes directly to the liver. Lymphatic fluid bathes our tissues in a pale, coagulable fluid. This fluid, riddled with toxins, is then distributed into the blood by way of the thoracic duct. Lymphatic massage allows excess fluids to flow into the lymph filtering stations to flush waste matter, preventing or minimizing escape into the bloodstream.

According to nutritionist Robert Gray, stimulating the lymph system with massage allows sticky mucoid toxic substances to be dumped into the colon for elimination, since the colon is the principal organ through which mucoid matter from the lymph is eliminated.

Dr. Loren Berry, one of the greatest of all manipulative healers, taught a technique of lymph drainage using massage therapy, although it was not widely accepted by traditional medical practitioners.

Dr. Olszewski of Poland conducted studies using scientific instruments capable of stimulating body surfaces by lymphatic massage and skin brushing. His studies concluded that the lymph undergoes *retrograde flow,* flow in the direction opposite to that which is considered normal. Also discovered is chylous reflux, a specific type of retrograde flow. Chylous reflux occurs when lymph flows from the *cisterna chyli* (the central lymphatic pool, in the abdomen) back into the colon or other body tissues.

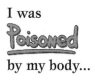

If the colon cannot perform the necessary purification of the lymph, the liver does the work instead. This adds toxic load for an already overworked liver, especially in digestive disorders.

When toxins are produced in the body at a faster rate than the body can process, the body protects us by suspending those toxins in fat and interstitial spaces in the attempt to protect organs. This excessive amount of toxins results in inflammation and excessive buildup of lymphatic fluids, as in fibromyalgia.

➤Flashback➤

When my thoracic area was swollen, it not only caused acute specific pain, but inflammation of the surrounding tissues. The medical diagnosis was "thoracic outlet syndrome." There was no medical explanation for the cause of the swelling or fluid buildup. Anti-inflammatory drug therapy and standard physical therapy were suggested and prescribed. Standard physical therapy brought me no relief; it included traditional massage and body mechanics, and no attention to the lymphatics. After my first lymphatic massage, the swelling was gone. It would gradually re-occur and after a lymphatic massage would again disappear. Finally, the body rid itself of enough toxins to facilitate the eventual elimination of swelling and pain.

There are several lymphatic drainage techniques. During this stage of my therapy, the therapist employed the Loren Berry method. The principles of his technique were developed from ancient Chinese medicine. The lymphatic massage therapist works from the colon to the periphery of the body, or from the center out. Space is thus created for the lymph fluid to drain. Undulating hand movements and specific compression are applied to move the fluid, allowing it to be carried through the lymph system and eliminated by the colon. The swelling is immediately reduced.

➤ Flashback ➤

There came a time when my body let my therapist and me know it no longer could handle a full session (1–1¹/₂ hours) of lymph drainage massage. When my body was detoxifying too quickly, I experienced accelerated fatigue and malaise. Subsequently, my therapist worked only on specific areas, for short periods of time, and with minimal pressure.

You *must* listen to your body, know your limits, and communicate with your therapist. If the massage is too intense, the resulting healing crises will cause you alarm and lack of trust in the therapist and therapy technique. Our bodies change daily as we detoxify. Have the therapist start out slowly with minimum stimulating pressure. Do *not* allow a therapist to talk you into a deeper massage than

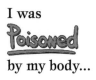
you can comfortably tolerate. You'll not only be in pain, but it can trigger an allergic response. For maximum benefit, the therapist must work at your speed to inspire trust, relaxation, and reduction of symptoms.

Castor Oil Packs: Lymphatic Value

Topical applications of castor oil are recommended by respected physician and researcher, Dr. William McGarey, for disturbances of the digestive system, including stomach, intestines, and colon. Dr. McGarey also recommends applications of castor oil for problems of the kidney, liver, and gall bladder. His work, in cooperation with the Association for Research and Enlightenment, confirms the use of castor oil for disturbances in the lymphatic, circulatory, urinary, and excretory systems. Castor oil has numerous external applications and can be applied by massaging the oil into the skin or by applying castor oil packs. I find castor oil extremely valuable for reducing the inflammation of both the abdominal area and liver region.

Castor oil increases the activity and movement of lymph fluid through the vessels. By increasing mobility of the lymphatic system, fats and other waste deposits are eliminated more quickly. Physical activity, massage stimulation, and application of castor oil encourage circulation of lymph.

According to Dr. McGarey castor oil absorbed in the tissues stimulates the parasympathetic nerve system, located in the area being treated. This, in turn, stimulates the lymphatics to more adequately drain the tissues under stress. Such activity would be beneficial to any organ or portion of the body clogged with waste products.

Food Elimination/Challenge Plan

Charting the Challenger

The consumption reaction connection (CRC) method of testing was one of the first types used for allergy reactive patients. It involves recording what you consume and the reactions you experience. CRC testing assists in making a connection to the offending substances. War on allergens begins with a strategy of attack by first identifying the enemy. It should be executed under the care of a nutritionally aware health-care practitioner. One of the most helpful suggestions I can share is to record *everything* you consume in a diary. Be careful to read labels so every ingredient is identified. When a reaction occurs, knowing specifically what you consumed provides a starting point for the CRC. By doing this exercise you'll be helping yourself and your health-care practitioner identify the causes of your reactions.

Sample charts shown on the following pages, if filled out precisely, will assist in identifying the offending substances.

FOOD ROTATION / REACTION CHART

	(Date) Day 1	Foods Consumed	Day 2	Foods Consumed
BREAKFAST				
Reaction				
SNACK				
Reaction				
LUNCH				
Reaction				
SNACK				
Reaction				
DINNER				
Reaction				
SNACK				
Reaction				

FOOD ROTATION

FOOD ROTATION / REACTION CHART

	Day 3	Foods Consumed	Day 4	Foods Consumed
BREAKFAST				
Reaction				
SNACK				
Reaction				
LUNCH				
Reaction				
SNACK				
Reaction				
DINNER				
Reaction				
SNACK				
Reaction				

FOOD ROTATION

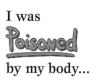
Food Elimination /Challenge Reintroduction Plan

When food allergies exist or are suspected, a basic elimination diet is the best approach. In patients such as myself, with severe reactions leading to anaphylactic shock, it is a critical first step. I suggest starting with a modified fast of fresh juices, brown rice, and quinoa, supplemented with a medical-food-quality rice protein-based drink. I used three formulas in my overall therapy. One is pure organic brown rice protein powder made by NutriBiotic™. This product adds only rice protein and no additional nutritional support. However, sometimes it's necessary to start as basic as plain organic rice protein for a couple of weeks, until other foods can be tolerated.

As my tolerance allowed, I began alternating between two other products that provide protein and supporting nutrients: Goatein™ from Garden of Life and BioInflammatory® by BioGenesis. They are available through health-care providers (see product resources). Goatein™ is a balanced combination of whey and milk proteins that contain no antibiotics or female growth hormones. Goatein™ contains powerful probiotics and naturally occurring digestive enzymes contributing to the health of the digestive tract while assisting overall absorption. Additionally, it contains a full compliment of easily absorbed amino acids for optimal health. Goat's milk protein is substantially less allergenic and easier to digest than cow's milk protein because the smaller molecules are closer in size and composition to human milk. Goatein™ is partially pre-digested through a lactic acid fermentation process to make it bio-available and virtually *lactose free.*

BioInflammatory® is a medical food formulated with rice flour and specialty anti-inflammatory nutrients to reduce inflammation, promote repair of damaged tissues and assist in liver detox. It is well tolerated in acutely sensitive patients until sufficient detoxification has taken place to allow for animal type proteins.

At the onset of my allergic reactions and anaphylactic shock, I followed a diet of fresh juice combinations (listed below), brown rice products (including bread, crackers, cereal), and rice milk, with added rice protein medical food. Any diet regime should be under the guidance of a healthcare professional. Do not attempt an elimination diet plan on your own.

Fresh juices are high in vitamins and especially enzymes. I recommend starting with the following combinations. Remember to start with two or three ingredients so you can chart any adverse reactions. These combinations will help the digestive system rest, start the detoxification process, and heal.

- Carrot, apple, and ginger ▪ Carrot, celery, and ginger ▪ Carrot, parsley, celery, and ginger ▪ Carrot, apple, parsley, ginger, broccoli stems, or any green vegetable tolerated ▪ Carrot, parsley, beets, apple, celery, ginger

If the concentrated juice causes any stomach distress, dilute with equal parts of pure water.

As you improve and cleanse your liver and

colon, fasting on these juices one to two days a week will help speed the healing process of the digestive tract by giving it a vacation. Be sure to check with your physician or health-care practitioner before starting any fasting program.

Start with a simple diet of the low-stress foods mentioned above. After two weeks, begin to add other low-allergy ingredients to both your juice and individual foods. For example, if you've been drinking juice made with carrots, apples, and ginger, you can now add beets, parsley, and so forth. If you've been consuming quinoa, add brown rice or an egg (assuming you don't have an allergy to eggs). Make sure to chart how you feel and look for symptoms of headache, sleeplessness, abdominal bloating, gas, or any other allergic reaction. If any items introduced seem to evoke a symptom, eliminate them and see if you notice any improvement.

The following charts are provided as guides for slowly reintroducing foods that are best tolerated in a program of continued detoxification.

As your condition improves through detoxification and repair, your body will produce more digestive enzymes. With more naturally occurring enzymes, the food is better digested before being absorbed, thus decreasing the severity of allergic reactions. Keep in mind that all people with leaky gut have Candida and/or parasites. Therefore, following a strict diet of eliminating all sugars and sugar-containing foods to starve the Candida, and a cleansing program for parasites, is imperative to overall healing.

LEAKY GUT—FOOD REINTRODUCTION PROGRAM

Consume all foods as tolerated

VEGETABLES	MEAT AND EGGS	FATS, OILS, & NUTS	STARCH/GRAINS
Beet Tops	Organic Eggs	Avocado	Brown Basmati Rice
Beets		Finely Ground Almonds	Brown Rice
Broccoli		Ghee	Brown Rice Bread
Carrot		Olive Oil	Brown Rice Cakes
Celery		Organic Real Butter	Brown Rice Chips (eden)
Chives		Safflower Oil	Brown Rice Crackers
Garlic		Sesame Seed Oil	Cream of Rice
Green Peas		Sunflower Oil	Quinoa
Leeks			Rice Cereal
Onions			Rice Pancakes
Pumpkin			Rice Pasta
Snow Peas			Tapioca
Spaghetti Squash			Teff
Spinach			
String Beans			
Summer Squash			
Swiss Chard			
Winter Squash		All food may be sweetened with Stevia (a natural sweetener)	
Yams		Foods should not contain artificial colors.	
Zucchini			

CHEESE AND DAIRY	SOUPS	BEVERAGES
Almond Cheese	Homemade Vegetarian Soups	Almond Milk
Goat Milk Products	Vegetable based broths	Berry Juice (No Seeds or Sugar)
Organic Goats Milk	Vegetarian Chicken Broth	Chamomile Tea
Rice Cheese		Fennel Tea
		Ginger Tea
		Non-citrus herb teas
HERBS/SPICES	**FRUIT**	Organic Coffee (2 cups a day)
		Rice Carob Milk
Apple Mint	Apples	Rice Milk
Barage	Cantaloupe(wash skin thoroughly)	Slippery Elm Tea
Basil	Grapes (In moderation)	Unsweetened fruit juice
Bayleaf	Guava (In moderation)	Unsweetened vegetable juice
Cilantro	Kiwi	(All Juices Should Be Bottled)
Coriander	Melons (well washed)	
Lavender	Organic Apple Sauce (glass)	
Mint	Organic Plum Sauce (glass)	
Parsley	Plum/Prune Plums (Fresh)	
Rosemary	Unsweetened Applesauce	
Saffron	Watermelon	
Sage	Berries (seedless puree or jelly)	
Tarragon		
Thyme		
Turmeric		

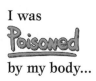
━Flashback━

At the onset of my disease, it was impossible to focus on any specific diet. The modified-fast diet became my basic safe standby. Survival was foremost. Fresh juices contain natural-occurring sugars that feed the Candida. However, the benefits of live enzymes from fresh juice outweigh the sugar factor. I did eliminate all other sugar and sugar-containing foods.

Most of my clients with chronic digestive and inflammatory disorders benefit from this elimination/challenge program. Clients who first resisted the program eventually gave it a try, after succumbing to other methods and medications with no relief. The results were twofold: reduction or elimination of the allergic symptoms and help in identifying the offending food.

Food Rotation Plan

In this dietary plan you rotate foods, so every day for five days you consume only certain vegetables, grains, fruits, and sources of protein, as tolerated. The following foods are the largest contributors of food allergies, and should be avoided:

- Wheat
- Eggs
- Peanuts
- Dairy
- Yeast
- Gluten-containing foods

After five days, the cycle begins again, so what you eat on Day One you can eat again on Day Six, and what you eat on Day Two you can repeat on Day Seven. This system allows a full four days without repeating a food.

If a little is good, repetition can trigger a reaction.

By rotating foods you are calling on only certain enzyme systems on that day, allowing other systems a chance to recover. Also, like the elimination diet, the rotation dietary plan makes it easy for you to see which foods are causing problems. It is important to eat a variety of foods; however, those of us with LGS can't always include all food groups. After you start detoxifying and healing, you'll be able to regain tolerance to previously allergic foods.

If you identify and eliminate an allergic food for four to six weeks or longer, you can possibly reintroduce it again, but in small quantities and on a rotated schedule. This way your body won't be as prone to again lose tolerance for the food. It is very important to maintain rotation for *everything* you consume, including protein drinks and medical food supplements.

These recommendations are a primary tool, not cast in concrete, for those of us challenged by leaky gut.

➤ Flashback ➤

I was so excited when I had my first batch of organic, creamy, smooth, homemade goat cheese that I ate it several times a day for several days. On about the seventh day, my throat closed and I had a full-blown reaction again.

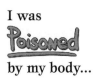
The significance of the seventh day of the week should have been my first clue. I didn't allow my digestive system to rest from the newly introduced food, so I got stopped in my tracks. I was so discouraged. My body not only needed the protein, it craved it! After two weeks of abstinence, I reintroduced the same type of cheese, with no problems. Now I eat my delicious protein on a rotational diet.

The following books are excellent resources for allergy and rotational diets. They would be beneficial as you introduce new and unusual foods and combinations.

The Allergy Self-Help Cookbook; Marjorie Jones, R.N., Rodale Press, 1984

5 Years without Food—The Food Allergy Survival Guide; Nicolette Dumke, Adapt Books, 1998

If This is Tuesday, It Must Be Chicken; Natalie Golos and Frances Golos Golbitz, Keats Publishing, 1983

Allergy & Candida Cooking Made Easy; Sondra Lewis, Canary Connect Publications, 1996

Organic Gourmet; Leslie Cerier, Station Hill Openings-Barrytown, Ltd., 1996

Dietary Life-Style Changes

Water, Water, Water

If you do not drink enough water during a cleansing and detoxifying routine, you will endanger the health of your tissues because concentrated toxins are being eliminated from your cells and colon. Our body is approximately 70 percent water. The body's water supply is responsible for running the systems of digestion, absorption, circulation, and elimination. Replacing the water continually lost through sweat and elimination is crucial. Water is so critical, and dehydration can have such damaging effects that lack of it can lead to death. The body can survive without food for approximately four to six weeks; however, without water it can only exist for about five days.

I find it very helpful to drink water out of a sipper bottle with a built-in straw. I have a 32-ounce sipper bottle in every location: car, office, and home. Somehow the sipping action allows us to consume larger amounts effortlessly. If you have chemical sensitivities, be cautious of plastic and use glass instead. Dr. Batmanghelidj, author of *Your Body's Many Cries for Water*, recommends drinking *half of your body weight in ounces.* For example, if you weigh 160 pounds, you need to consume eighty ounces of water each day (equal to ten cups). If you weigh 200 pounds, then drink one hundred ounces of water each day (equal to 12½ cups).

Clients report that, although challenging at first, within two weeks their body is craving more water. Drinking pure water allows your body to flush out the toxins without having to mobilize the digestive system. Caffeine-free tea, hot or cold, counts for part of your daily intake. However, be careful with some herbal teas containing ingredients with stimulating effects; they make your body systems work instead of resting and restoring. Drinking water with some fresh lemon is beneficial for most healthy people; however, with leaky gut, citrus can cause disturbing reactions. It is best to get into a routine of just plain, pure water, water, water.

Organic Food, a Necessary Choice

There are 1,500,000,000 pounds of pesticides used in the United States each year on agricultural food products. This amounts to nearly five pounds of poisonous sprays for each person. About 45,000 different agricultural chemicals are used and one hundred fifty of these regularly appear as residue in food, with about two dozen of them at toxic levels.

If the bugs won't eat these chemicals, why should we?

Why subject yourself and your family to the effects of these chemicals, when you can purchase or grow organic foods? Yes, it takes some planning, but don't wait until your reactions reach the level of anaphylactic shock before you change your choice of foods and their source. Make sure produce is labeled "Certified Organically Grown." This is the best assurance that the food is truly organic. Anything less is questionable. Organic foods bring us health, not disease. They generally cost more than conventionally grown food, but as powerfully stated by Leslie Cerier, author of *The Organic Gourmet,* organic foods are "the cheapest health insurance around for you, your family, and the environment."

Our bodies were not engineered to process synthetic substances.

➤ Flashback ➤

*Every time I had non-organic food, I reacted within
twelve to fifteen minutes. When consuming the same
foods certified organic, I experienced no reaction.
Now my entire diet consists of only organic foods.*

Smaller, More Frequent Meals

For a person with severe allergic reactions and
with a toxic colon, it is essential to nourish the body
frequently and in smaller portions. This way of eating
is not unlike a routine diabetic diet: small amounts of
food every $1^1/_2$ to $2^1/_2$ hours. It's important to keep
the body nourished and blood-sugar levels neutral,
while not overworking the digestive system.

➤ Flashback ➤

*For the first few weeks, I had fresh juice at
alternating intervals with brown rice. I set a timer
on my desk to remind me to eat every $1^1/_2$ hours. If I
got busy and didn't eat within that time, the
reaction was the same as if I had eaten an allergic
food. At times I ate grated carrots or apples and
fresh applesauce as a snack. As I improved, I
extended the time between eating to $2^1/_2$–3 hours.*

I believe my body reacted the same to an empty
stomach as to foods it couldn't tolerate because the
toxins from the leaky gut were circulating through my
system without being diluted by digestion of food. I
also noticed that every time a reaction occurred on an
empty stomach and colon hydrotherapy was administered, the reaction stopped.

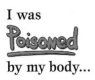
Supplementing Minerals "My Whey"

We Are Electrical Creatures

Minerals are the body's electrical transmitter. They serve as electrical signals to every cell. Brain signals are transmitted through body fluids. Intestinal disorders, particularly leaky gut, cause a deficiency of minerals.

There are two groups of minerals, macro-minerals (bulk) and micro-minerals (trace).

- **Macro-minerals** include calcium, magnesium, sodium, potassium, and phosphorus. For proper electrical transmission, the body needs these minerals in larger amounts than trace minerals. Muscle cramping and pain are common symptoms in inflammatory and intestinal disorders. These symptoms are usually the result of unbalanced minerals. The deficiency can also occur as a result of excessive consumption of water, dietary salt, some prescription drugs, and colon irrigation.

- **Micro-minerals** include zinc, iron, copper, manganese, chromium, selenium, and iodine. These minerals are needed in only minute quantities; however, they are critical for balanced health and healing.

Minerals are stored primarily in the body's bone and muscle tissue. The absorbed mineral must be carried by the blood to the cells and then absorbed by the cell membrane to be utilized by the cell. When the mineral enters the body through the intestinal lining, it competes with other minerals for absorption; therefore, minerals should always be taken in balanced proportions.

Examples of Mineral Imbalances

Excessive consumption of:	*Causes depletion of:*
Zinc	Copper and Iron
Calcium	Magnesium and Zinc
Copper	Zinc
Phosphorus	Calcium

A product that does an exceptional job in mineral replacement and supplementation in Capra Mineral Whey Powder®, manufactured by Mt. Capra Cheese Company. It is a mineral-rich, golden brown, dry natural food powder from dehydrated organic goat milk whey. Absorbability is always an important consideration with leaky gut and intestinal disorders. For this reason, this form of mineral supplementation has shown superior reduction or elimination of symptoms, with a greater absorption factor than tablets or capsules.

Capra Mineral Whey® was first introduced to me by my colon hydotherapist. It provides excellent mineral supplementation after colon therapy. It can be taken cold in water or juice, or as a "hot toddy" in boiling water.

The powder is grainy but very sweet and tasty. I recommend anyone using enemas or colon hydrotherapy to consider this product for mineral/electrolyte replacement. The most plentiful mineral ingredients in Capra Mineral Whey are electrolytes. These electrolytes make up the electrically charged ions that help transport and regulate water balance,

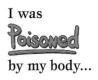
acid-alkaline balance, osmotic pressure, nerve impulse conduction, and muscle contraction into and out of the cells. Capra Mineral Whey® contains mineral combinations found in whole foods. Because of its high sodium, potassium, and calcium content, this whey has an alkaline reaction.

"My Whey"

"Whey to go!" It's amazing how quickly those "charley horses" went trotting off somewhere else, rather than over my legs.

Capra Mineral Whey Powder eliminated my muscle spasms and aches within three days of initial consumption. I took two tablespoons in a small amount of water or juice three times daily. After several months, I reduced the amount to two tablespoons, once daily. If muscle spasms reoccur, I increase the amount for a few days until symptoms are eliminated. When spasms reoccur after disappearing, it is important to determine what changed in the daily routine to cause depletion of minerals. Possible causes are excessive sweating, frequent colon irrigation (more than once a week), excessive intake of carbonated drinks, and diarrhea.

Fiber *decreases* absorption of minerals, so take supplemental fiber or bulking agents at different times. It is best, but not always possible, to wait 4-6 hours between mineral supplementation and fiber-bulking agents. For example, take fiber-bulking agents at bedtime and mineral supplementation in the morning. If two doses of minerals are needed, take one upon rising and another in late afternoon or early evening.

I used a colloidal, organic, liquid-mineral supplementation before developing leaky gut. Afterward, I couldn't take it without experiencing a reaction. After researching and comparing ingredients, I concluded that most colloidal mineral combinations contained citric acid, not well tolerated by a compromised gut.

Another Essential Goat Milk Product: Goatein™

The nutritional analysis of goats' milk shows it to be exceptional. It is high in natural amino acids and minerals and contains some vitamins. Animal protein (such as Goatein™) is the *only* source of complete protein available. Its distinct advantage over vegetarian sources (such as soy) is that they are typically low in one or more of the essential amino acids—even when overall protein content is high. Other research confirms that milk protein is also superior to rice, wheat and beef for quality and overall bioavailablilty. Goatein™, made by Garden of Life, is the highest quality protein powder available because it's processed without the use of acid or excessive heat. This process allows the amino acids, enzymes, and beneficial bacteria to remain in their natural form—making it my protein powder of choice. Colon function thrives when provided with whole, human-grade goat milk protein, which is a natural, ideal food to promote the growth of healthy colon flora.

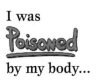
Nutritional Support and
Vitamin Supplementation

Glutamine

Glutamine is an amino acid derived from the fermentation process of grain. It is then purified so as to eliminate any potential allergic reactions. Glutamine is a preferred fuel for the cells that make up your gastrointestinal tract, as well as for your immune system. This amino acid is primary energy fuel for the small intestine.

Glutamine is a nonessential amino acid, meaning that in a healthy person it is normally produced at a sufficient rate to adequately supply glutamine-consuming tissues. Of all the amino acids incorporated into protein, *glutamine is the most abundant in the human body.*

In the patient with nutritional depletion, common with food allergies, leaky gut, and intestinal disorders, decreased muscle tissue and changes in intermediary metabolism lead to diminished glutamine production. This depletion results in decreased availability and uptake of plasma glutamine concentration in the gut.

Laboratory studies show that parts of the immune system (especially liver and spleen) switch from release of glutamine to consumption of glutamine after a trauma. The hypothesis is that in a depleted state, such as loss of muscle mass, the capacity to produce sufficient glutamine for the immune system is diminished. As a consequence of diminished availability of glutamine, a deterioration of the gut mucosal barrier is expected.

The digestive tract uses glutamine not only as a fuel source, but also for healing stomach ulcers, irritable bowel syndrome, ulcerative bowel diseases, and leaky gut syndrome. It is also used to soothe the digestive tract in celiac patients. Glutamine is the most popular anti-ulcer drug in Asia today. Basically, glutamine helps heal the leaky cells and is a fuel source that facilitates healing of the digestive tract. Check with your nutritionally-aware physician or health-care practitioner for therapy guidelines.

Glutamine is also important for the health of the intestinal mucosa. Recent studies show that glutamine helps maintain healthy muscle tissue by regulating muscle protein synthesis. In fact, glutamine appears to be the most important amino acid for regulating protein synthesis. In addition, when the body and its immune system is stressed and glutamine is in short supply, the body borrows directly from muscle tissue, breaking it down to use as energy. Supplementing the body's natural supply of glutamine short-circuits the body's need to borrow from its own muscle tissue. Lost muscle tone is especially evident in inflammatory disorders such as fibromyalgia.

Glutamine also helps maintain healthy glutathione (GSH) levels. Glutathione is considered by many experts to be the most important antioxidant produced by the body.

The goal of glutamine supplementation is to diminish damage to your GI tract, decrease symptoms, and enhance the antioxidant and immune response systems. As a bonus, glutamine supports healthy brain function and is considered "brain fuel." Anyone suffering the consequences of LGS,

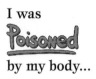
MCSS/EI, and digestive disorders appreciates any brain fuel we can get!

Supplementation with glutamine is essential in LGS and digestive disorders. BioInflammatory medical food powder provides 1000 mg. of glutamine along with supporting nutrients for detoxification of metabolic waste products and environmental toxins, such as: heavy metals, pesticides, herbicides, solvents, drug residues, etc.

Ginger: A Natural Digestive Aid

Ginger root (*Zingiber officicinale*) is an ancient herb used extensively for thousands of years in Chinese, Ayurvedic, and Western healing modalities. It tastes good in food, as a stimulating and warming tea, or in fresh juices. Ginger is especially beneficial in cases of exhaustion from chronic disease because it strengthens the entire body. Cleansing heals, but also puts stress on the digestive system. Ginger helps neutralize the stress of detoxifying. Because of its anti-inflammatory properties, ginger assists in pain management while reducing gas, indigestion, and nausea. Studies show that ginger is at least as effective as prescription drugs for general nausea and motion sickness, without the possible side effects. I recommend using ginger in cooking, stir-fry, and particularly in fresh juice (see recipes in "Food Elimination/Challenge Reintroduction Plan").

Some of the benefits of ginger:
- Cleanses the colon, stomach, small intestine, circulatory system, and liver
- Stimulates circulation

- Reduces spasms
- Reduces muscle cramps
- Increases bile secretion
- Provides antioxidant protection for the liver
- Has antibacterial properties
- Provides anti-parasitic properties to assist in eliminating worms
- Protects the heart by lowering cholesterol and inhibiting platelet aggregation
- Normalizes bowel function
- Restores colon tone

Aloe Vera Juice

As far back as I can remember, I was told about the miraculous benefits of the aloe vera plant. Raised by my paternal grandmother, a natural herbalist, it was impossible for me to avoid learning about herbs. I remember aloe vera growing on our patio in southern California. Every time someone had a skin burn or digestive heartburn, grandma ran out to pluck a leaf. As a child, I accepted most of this information as "old wives' tales," only to find out later what has been proven for centuries: your house isn't complete if aloe vera isn't growing in your patio or kitchen window.

Now scientific research attests to the boundless powers of aloe vera doing exactly what the "old wives' tales" proclaimed:

- Eases the pain and heals wounds caused by searing, scalding, sunburn, radiation, and other types of burns.
- Heals skin ulcerations, relieves dermatitis, seborrhea, and acne.

- Proves effective against peptic ulcers and oral ulcers.
- Cleanses infections and retards fungus growth.
- Provides superior and totally natural cosmetic benefits.
- Has a natural laxative effect.

These are documented matters of record regarding use of aloe vera. The results are published in some of the most prestigious scientific journals and textbooks of medical literature. The aloe plant was used by ancient civilizations and given the common name of Curacao or Barbados Aloe, suggesting a New World origin. However, aloe vera is native to the Mediterranean region of southern Europe and North Africa. Using the juice of the aloe plant as a cathartic (laxative) goes back to the early days of Greece and Rome. The plant was introduced into the Caribbean in the seventeenth century to be cultivated for its juice, which was then evaporated and exported back to Europe as a drug for constipation.

Aloe vera is a member of the lily family, but it does not resemble its distant cousin. Aloe vera is a perennial succulent that is drought-resistant. The outside skin of the leaf is smooth, fairly thick, with a rubbery texture. Right below the outside layer are the cells that secrete the juice used to make the drug aloe. The inner chamber is made up of the clear gel, or pulp, resembling slightly melted lemon Jell-O®. The pulp is believed to contain wound-healing agents, called "biogenic stimulators" by the Russians.

You can purchase aloe vera juice in health-food stores and pharmacies. It also comes in gel and capsules. There is a mild laxative element with some of the capsules, but not with the juice or gel. Be sure it contains at least 70 percent aloe vera.

The juice protects the mucous membranes and, therefore, has a healing and soothing effect on the digestive tract. In constipation or diarrhea it will assist in returning the stools to normal. In addition, I find aloe vera juice to be effective for food allergies and to protect the digestive system when it is necessary to take prescription drug medication. I routinely took 1 oz (a jigger full) of aloe vera juice and the effects were very calming to an angry stomach or gut.

Candida: Fighting Your Fungus

It's been widely reported that antibiotics change the balance of intestinal micro-flora. Antibiotics kill both beneficial and harmful bacteria throughout our body, especially in our digestive system. This creates the perfect condition for bacteria, parasites, viruses, and yeasts that are resistant to antibiotics. In a healthy intestinal tract, these harmful bacteria may be present in small numbers without any adverse reactions or symptoms. However, once the overgrowth occurs, they produce waste material that becomes poisonous chemicals to the cells and the body they live in. *Candida albicans* (yeast) is nothing new to the medical profession. As clearly stated by Dr. Ralph Golan, "At one extreme, it can cause skin rashes or vaginal infections (mucocutaneous candidiasis). At the other extreme, in individuals whose immune systems are severely compromised, yeast can invade the bloodstream (candidemia) and cause death." Your present leaky gut, and the accompanying *Candida*, may not yet have reached life-threatening proportions, but nonetheless present a major roadblock to healing.

In real estate it's been said that a piece of property is only as good as its location, location, location. In healing the leaky gut, managing and eliminating *Candida* is essential, and that effectiveness depends primarily on diet, diet, diet. The challenge for the leaky gut patient is that a typical *Candida* diet cannot be strictly followed due to the allergic reactions, gut consequences, and the resulting generalized malnutrition. Therefore, the following guidelines are provided in general terms to assist you in avoiding foods that directly contribute to yeast growth. The guidelines do not apply during the time of healing the leaky gut, unless your tolerance for foods is greater than previously indicated.

When these guidelines are strictly adhered to for six to twelve weeks, the body will suffocate or starve the yeast fungus. In some cases, there is an initial worsening of symptoms as the yeast die off (Herxheimer reaction), and the associated toxins circulate through the body. The yeast fungus eats first, and your body gets their leftovers, including toxic by-products of their digestion and the actual die-off. Colon cleansing at this phase of detoxification is essential. After about three weeks (be sure to check with your health-care practitioner), you should feel a relief of symptoms and renewed physical and emotional energy. Eliminating overgrowth of *Candida* requires a life-long commitment to eliminating sugars and sugar-forming foods.

What to Avoid

- Sugar and sugar-containing foods:

   Sugar is sugar, whether it's refined or unrefined, such as turbinado, dried cane juice, raw sugar, honey, maple syrup, or molasses. Be aware, read labels, because sugar comes in many disguises. *Candida* multiplies at an alarming rate in a sugary environment. Fruit, other than in fresh juices, should be limited to a daily maximum of one serving. Fruits contain mostly sugar, so limit yourself to a half piece of fruit for one serving or as many small fruits as will fit in the palm of your hand. One whole apple or half an apple and a small bunch of grapes would constitute your total daily allotment.

- Artificial Sweeteners:

   NutraSweet® and Equal® (aspartame) have been known to cause severe allergic reactions, both physically and psychologically.

   You can use Stevia, a natural herbal found in your health-food store. Stevia is two hundred times sweeter than sugar, so use caution. If you use more than minute amounts, it will be bitter. Stevia does not raise blood-sugar levels in the body or contribute to yeast growth. It is

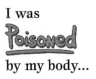
available in liquid or concentrated powder. I find the liquid extract much easier to use. For example: I use six to seven drops in a bowl of hot cereal, it's naturally healthy, powerful, and economical.

- Cheese and dairy:

   Avoid all processed and aged cheeses. Organic fresh goat cheese is acceptable in moderate amounts. Milk and milk products are simple carbohydrates, which feed the yeast.

- Yeast-containing foods:

   Avoid breads and pastries that are yeast-leavened.

   Alcoholic beverages

   Avoid beer and wine fermented and/or brewed with yeast.

- Gluten-containing grains:

   Avoid especially wheat, oats, rye, and barley.

- Fungi and moldy foods

   Avoid citric acid, truffles, morels, mushrooms. Tempeh is a white cultured mold closely related to the mushroom.

- Vinegar-containing foods:

   Avoid mustard, ketchup, steak sauces, barbecue sauces, green olives, horseradish, mayonnaise, pickles, and most salad dressings.

- Fermented products:

   Avoid root beer, cider, soy sauce, and tamari. It is acceptable to use Braggs Amino Acids®, a naturally fermented soy product that is a good replacement for traditional soy sauce. Miso is a fermented soybean product.

Caffeine-containing products:

Avoid coffee, tea, chocolate, and other foods containing caffeine. You can substitute carob for chocolate. Carob-flavored rice milk is a delicious substitute for chocolate milk.

■ Dried or canned fruits:

Dried fruits become a highly concentrated sugar and can collect mold during the drying process. Canned fruit is processed, and therefore should be avoided when possible.

Benefits of Garlic

To combat *Candida*, diet control is major; however, I also recommend additional supplements that assist in killing yeast faster. Garlic is one such natural supplement complementing your diet by killing off yeast overgrowth without the side effects of drugs. In leaky gut-type syndromes and the accompanying *Candida*, the addition of supplemental garlic speeds recovery, minimizing infections of the immune system.

In 1858, Louis Pasteur first proved garlic to be a natural antibiotic. His research demonstrated the ability of garlic to kill bacteria in laboratory culture dishes.

Dr. Benjamin Lau, famed immunologist, conducted experiments testing the ability of various potent drugs to stop the growth of bacteria and fungi. His findings proved garlic extract stopped the

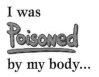
growth of those cultures even more effectively than the potent drugs being used for the same purpose. His research confirmed garlic to be a potent, broad-spectrum antibiotic and anti-fungal. His research also concluded that garlic worked particularly on the mold that causes *Candida albicans.* Garlic acts on the lipid layer of the cell membrane, interfering with lipid synthesis and with the yeast organism's ability to take up oxygen. In other words, garlic causes these microbes to lose their membrane, the lining of their bodies, and consequently they can no longer breathe. Studies confirmed what the Chinese have known for centuries: garlic inhibits viral multiplication.

According to research conducted in the Department of Microbiology at the University of Oklahoma, garlic juice is as effective as the anti-fungal drugs amphotericin and nystatin. Researchers confirmed the benefits of garlic, next came the challenge of producing *socially acceptable garlic,* without the taste and odor.

Garlic Supplementation

The beneficial constituent of garlic is the alliin. The higher the alliin count, the greater the benefit. Scientific studies presented at the World Garlic Conference (1990) stated categorically that cooked garlic and garlic extract in liquid or powdered form have the same properties as raw garlic.

Many good brands of garlic are on the market. Manufacturers of garlic capsules and tablets have successfully found a way of maintaining the alliin benefits without the taste and odor. You will, at times, detect the fragrance of garlic when opening a bottle in the supplemental form. However, this doesn't mean you will taste or smell like garlic. If you use a brand that does stimulate body odor, change brand. The difference in our body chemistry will not react the same to every composition.

I like the properties of Garlic 7000 by BioGenesis, available through health-care providers.

To receive long-term benefits, it is important for garlic to be supplemented daily, not as a random "quick fix." However, just as important as consistency is the correct amount of supplementation. Check with your health-care practitioner before starting supplementation. In LGS and digestive disorders, *excessive* supplemental garlic may cause destruction of the body's beneficial bacteria within the digestive tract. In *rare* cases, toxicity and swelling of the liver can occur if *raw* garlic is consumed in excessive amounts.

Liver Detoxification and Support

The liver is generally the organ that bears the burden of faulty digestion and leaky gut. In my case, liver symptoms included jaundice skin, yellowish color to whites of eyes, chronic swelling under right breast, and acute sharp pains. The following therapies and supportive supplements have been critical in my healing process.

It is important to cleanse the colon before embark-

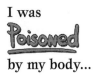
ing on a liver detoxification program. Colon cleansing reduces the amount of waste and toxins circulated through the liver, allowing the liver to start the repair process. Once a disease has been established as chronic, you must suspect suppressed liver detoxification. Although at times difficult to measure, liver toxicity adds up to the total amount of toxins and the ability to eliminate them. Ultimately, liver health predicts the overall health of the individual.

Homeopathic Support

A special complex formulated by Daystar Remedies provided me with natural support during and after the detoxification process. This comes in a liquid form and several drops are taken sublingually (under the tongue) as recommended by your health-care practitioner. More often than not with leaky gut, the homeopathic remedy provides gentle support without causing fast detoxification, triggering a reaction or liver pain. It is available through your health-care practitioner.

➤Flashback◄

For months, I could not tolerate any form of supplemental support for the liver except the homeopathic remedy by Daystar. When the liver became swollen, I would take as many as six drops every fifteen minutes until the pain subsided (usually after four to five doses). Today, long after the swelling is gone, I continue to take six drops morning and night for liver maintenance support.

Alfalfa Tablets

One of the richest mineral foods, alfalfa root, grows as far as 130 feet into the earth. Alfalfa contains chlorophyll, potassium, magnesium, iron, manganese, copper, calcium, phosphorus, and vitamins A, C, D, E, K, B1, B12, and niacin. The minerals are in a balanced form. Chlorophyll in alfalfa aids in the healing of intestinal ulcers, gastritis, liver disorders, hemorrhoids, constipation, poor body and breath odor, bleeding gums, infections, burns, athlete's foot, and cancer. Alfalfa tablets have all the fiber material from the stems and fiber structure of the alfalfa leaves. These act as bulk material to support a weakened bowel. This action allows for a faster transit time in the bowel. Alfalfa is one of the supplements I wouldn't be without.

In an extremely toxic bowel, you might experience additional gas. Alter the dose until no symptoms occur. This is usually a temporary condition and will improve as detoxification progresses. According to Dr. Bernard Jensen, the recommended maintenance supplementation is five tablets morning and evening. When my liver swelling was acute, I experienced a reduction of symptoms by taking five tablets three times daily.

Milk Thistle (Silybum marianum)

Milk thistle seed is a mild digestive bitter used in treating skin disorders and for cleansing the blood. Used since antiquity for digestive and liver complaints, it increases secretion and flow of bile. It gently promotes liver cleansing, but its primary actions go beyond what is known as one of the strongest liver herbs. It protects the liver with its antioxidant properties and rebuilds it by supporting RNA synthesis, necessary for protein synthesis. It stimulates the production of new liver cells and prevents formation of damaging leukotrienes.

Milk thistle also protects the kidneys. The toxins our liver neutralizes come from within us as well as from the outside world. During the cleansing process, the liver has extra work to do as toxins are released from body tissues into the blood and lymph. Milk thistle seed extract protects the liver cells as they neutralize toxins, bind to them, and dump them into the colon for elimination from the body. At the same time, milk thistle seed extract is working hard to rebuild damaged liver tissue.

The healing properties of *Silybum* have been studied extensively for decades, primarily in Europe. *Silybum* has been used successfully to treat patients with chronic hepatitis and cirrhosis; it is active against hepatitis-B virus, and shown to lower fat deposits in the liver of animals. Because of its effects on cleansing the blood, milk thistle is also used for treating skin disorders such as psoriasis and eczema.

The homeopathic formula contains *Silybum,* but is much easier to tolerate for some people than the herbal, especially when liver function is severely compromised.

Life Cannot be Sustained
Without Enzymes

*Healing the
Leaky Gut
Naturally:
Not Medicine
as Usual*

153

Enzymes are essential for proper functioning of our body. They are found in all living plant and animal matter. Their primary job is to maintain balanced body functions, digest food, and aid in the repair of tissue. Made up of proteins, the thousands of known enzymes play a critical role in virtually all body activities. *Life cannot be sustained without enzymes,* despite the presence of sufficient amounts of vitamins, minerals, water, and proteins. Scientists are unable to manufacture enzymes synthetically. Each enzyme has a very specific biochemical function in the body and no other enzyme can be substituted.

According to Dr. Howard F. Loomis, Jr., "It is the enzymes that are responsible for the vast majority of all the biochemical reactions that bring our foods to maturity or ripeness." Enzymes are energy, and energy is defined in high school physics textbooks as the "capacity to do work." Enzymes are the electrical connectors driving metabolic functions. *Enzymes do not perform the work; rather they are the conductors.*

The shape of each specific enzyme is so specialized it will initiate a reaction in only certain substances. Because enzymes are needed at various body sites, it is important they not be overworked. In an overworked system, production and efficiency are greatly reduced. A healthy body does its work of manufacturing enzymes, while maintaining the capacity of subsidizing its supply obtained from food.

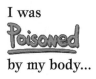
Unfortunately, enzymes are extremely sensitive to heat; even low temperatures will destroy enzymes. To obtain enzymes from a food source, the food must be eaten raw (as in fresh juice). Cooking or heating foods deplete all enzymes. So if your diet consists mostly of cooked food, you're lacking enzymes.

Digestive Enzymes

The primary work of digestive enzymes is to break down proteins, carbohydrates, and fats into smaller particles so the body can more easily absorb the nutrients through the stomach and small intestine. Digestion is primarily performed in the stomach and finished in the small intestine. The effect on intestinal micro-flora as a consequence of digestive efficiency includes stimulating the "good" bacteria in the gut, detoxifying and cleansing the colon, and improving digestive disorders, including food and environmental allergies.

The body contains over 3,000 types of enzymes. Many work in synchronicity with one another.

The primary enzymes used for digestion include:

- Proteases: break down proteins (beef, chicken, poultry, fish)
- Amylases: break down carbohydrates, including starches (bread, pasta, potatoes, fruits, vegetables, sugars)
- Cellulase: break down cellulose (plant fiber), the indigestible part of fiber found in many fruits and vegetables

- Lipase: break down fats
- Papain (proteolytic enzyme): break down proteins
- Bromelain (proteolytic enzyme): break down proteins
- Maltase: break down malt sugar, grains
- Lactase: break down milk sugar
- Invertase: break down sucrose (table sugar)

I alternate between two combinations very effectively, as do my clients, VegiZyme® by BioGenesis® and Zygest® from PhysioLogics®. Alternating is important to keep the body from rejecting the substance after a prolonged period of consumption. This also assists digestion in the best possible way by selectively choosing the combination that suits the meal being consumed. For protein or hard to digest foods, I take one high potency VegiZyme® because it contains three types of Protease that specifically assist in protein digestion: Protease, Protease II, Protease III. For other meals, two Zygest® prove effective. If you experience heartburn or indigestion at any time, especially at bedtime, take an additional one to two capsules of VegiZyme®. Usually the symptoms are eliminated within 15 minutes. Your healthcare provider will provide individual guidance for product use and dosage.

Note: Take digestive enzymes at the start of, or during, a meal.

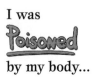
Systemic Oral Enzymes

Metabolic enzymes are used for systemic purposes in the bloodstream, unlike digestive enzymes that are used in the stomach and small intestine. Metabolic enzymes must be absorbed into the bloodstream in order to be effective. Enzymes made for systemic or metabolic functions are coated with an acid-resistant substance to prevent them from dissolving in an acid stomach. The next section provides an in-depth look at systemic metabolic enzymes and their uses.

Note: Take systemic enzymes *on an empty stomach,* at least 45 minutes before or after eating.

"I Hurt All Over": The Drug Alternative for Pain and Inflammation

When our bodies are unable to deal with toxic overload, the reaction is pain and inflammation. Many illnesses, and nearly all injuries, result in inflammatory reactions to various degrees. *There is a common denominator in leaky gut: inflammatory disorders and immune system dysfunction.* This is evident in related conditions such as fibromyalgia, chronic fatigue, lupus, arthritis, and myofascial pain syndrome. It is estimated that 26 million people, in the U.S. alone, have fibromyalgia, myofascial pain syndrome, or both. That figure is alarming to me, and it should be to you.

When the immune system malfunctions and becomes hyperactive, it overreacts and produces antibodies that attack even harmless substances in the blood. This causes formation of irritating circulating immune complexes (CICs), that are so misshapen and foreign to the body, they themselves are attacked by the immune system. Otherwise healthy tissues, in the same neighborhood, may also be impacted, causing further exacerbation of the immune reaction or response. This causes the immune system to attack both its own cells and the tissues of the body; the result, chronic pain and inflammation.

Most conventional treatments address symptoms of inflammation with anti-inflammatory medications, and don't address the underlying systemic condition. These medications reduce pain and inflammation but cause dangerous side effects and do nothing to start the healing process. I know— I've Done That Already (IDTA)!

Systemic oral enzymes stimulate healthy production of messenger immune cells (cytokines). These reduce inflammation and speed up immunity by producing a cleansing effect and helping to break up CICs at the center of the body's immune/inflammation reaction. The treatment of a disturbed or compromised immune system, however, requires patience and time. The effects of systemic oral enzyme therapy on the immune system and treatment of autoimmune diseases, especially rheumatoid factors, are profound, and may involve intense therapy for weeks or months. Remember, we're dealing with the causes of the disorder, *not suppressing or masking* the symptoms. If you're in acute pain, your physician can assist you in incorporating

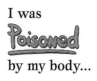
prescription drugs (for immediate relief) with enzyme therapy (for long-term healing).

Benefits of Metabolic/Systemic Oral Enzymes:

- Degrade protein molecules that penetrate from the blood capillaries into the tissues, where they subsequently cause edema and exacerbate the inflammatory process.
- Increase the flexibility of red blood cells, improving their ability to pass through the capillaries.
- Inhibit the aggregation of platelets.
- Degrade cell fragments and mediators of inflammation and infection.
- Increase the fibrinolytic activities in the blood, helping to prevent abnormal clotting.
- Activate white blood cells (macrophages) the natural killer cells, better equipping the immune system to deal with inflammation by cleansing itself of cellular debris and quickly neutralizing errant cancer cells.
- Support the cleansing of the tissues and promote better circulation.
- Stimulate formation of new, healthy tissue.

Enzyme therapy markedly reduces the body's inflammation level, enabling the person to once again resume normal activity and restore quality of life, naturally.

I reviewed hundreds of pages on systemic oral enzymes and used several dozen brands. The one product that is responsible for eliminating my chronic muscle pain and inflammation is Wobenzym®N, manufactured in Germany by the Mucos Pharma GmbH & Co. Recent research confirms it is now recognized as the #1 most effective oral enzyme in the world. Wobenzym®N is endorsed by leading European scientists and is backed by over thirty years of scientific research and clinical studies confirming its benefits.

Why hasn't my health-care provider recommended metabolic oral enzymes instead of drugs with their side effects?

Sadly, health-care providers may not know about systemic oral enzymes. Most European studies are not totally validated as a basis for clinical opinion in the U.S. Our medical education system tends to not teach nutrition; it teaches only the bare basics about the use of vitamin and mineral therapies. Most American medical journals have, until recently, avoided articles on nutrition, feeling they should be published elsewhere or not at all. It appears that a great majority of doctors seem uncomfortable recommending a food or natural substance rather than drugs. But this position is beginning to change. Our economy is now global, as are our resources for products. Multi-national clinical trials are now becoming more abundant. The information on medicine and therapies is now as close as your computer. The European research is as good, if not better, than the research done in America. It is my opinion that systemic oral enzymes offer the first mainstream long-term treatment option

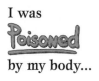
for inflammatory disorders, with proven healing and safety. This is particularly true when compared to corticosteroids and non-steroidal anti-inflammatory drugs (NSAIDs) with their side effects, of which I am a prime example.

I began by taking ten Wobenzym®N tablets three times a day on an empty stomach. The tablets are about the size of a commonly recognized round, candy-coated chocolate, without the coloring agent. The results were the same as when I took the NSAIDs. I now take a maintenance dose of five tablets three times a day. My clients report similar results and keep saying, "Why didn't someone tell me about systemic enzymes before now?" You be the judge. Wobenzym®N is available through health-care practitioners and select pharmacies.

Other Options for Managing Pain and Inflammation

Another product that enhances relief from pain and inflammation is BioInflammatory® capsules by BioGenesis®. This product is similar to the medical food in power form, except here only the specialty nutrients are included to effectively neutralize and remove free radical inflammatory agents. This method provides all the anti-inflammatory ingredients without the balanced caloric benefit of the medical food powder.

The second product is BioCleanse® by Bio-Genesis®. It is a medical food in powder form and specifically designed to remove toxins from your

Healing the
Leaky Gut
Naturally:
Not Medicine
as Usual

161

nervous system, connective and fatty tissues—therefore managing pain and inflammation. After the removal of toxins, BioCleanse® assists your liver in neutralizing and removing them from your body, through Phase 1 and Phase 2 pathways. It is a balanced formula of protein, carbohydrate and fats to maintain healthy blood sugar levels and energy. It provides 14 grams of protein per serving. It can be mixed with rice or nut milk to provide nourishment, pain relief, and minimize rapid weight loss. Your healthcare provider will guide you as to the product and dosage for your individual needs.

Parasites: Eliminating Your Unwanted Houseguests

You may be shocked to know what medical experts say about parasites:

"85% of adult North Americans are infected with parasites."

Dr. Hazel Parcels

"In terms of numbers, there are more parasitic infections acquired in this country than in Africa."

Dr. Frank Nova, Chief of the Laboratory for Parasitic Diseases of the U.S. National Institute of Health

"I believe the single most undiagnosed health challenge in the history of the human race is parasites."

Dr. Ross Anderson

It is my experience that most people with gastrointestinal disorders, inflammatory diseases, (such as arthritis and fibromyalgia), and allergies have parasites. This is especially evident in cases of leaky gut and irritable bowel syndrome. Most people falsely believe they do not have to concern themselves with the possibility of parasites if they haven't visited another country or traveled far from home. Nothing could be further from the truth. According to a report published by The Environmental Working Group in Washington, D.C., most municipal water systems in the U.S. are homes to protozoa like *Giardia* and *Cryptosporidium.* The group also reported that one in five Americans drinks water that violates federal health standards. Every year, nearly a million North Americans become sick from waterborne diseases; about 1 percent dies.

The type of worms living in the gastrointestinal tract includes tapeworm, threadworm, roundworm, pinworm, and hookworm.

Treatment for removal of parasitic infection is not a do-it-yourself project. There are many forms of natural therapies that do not have the side effects of drug therapies. One important fact to keep in mind, however, is that repeated therapies are sometimes required to achieve complete success. If you have a prolonged digestive disorder, you should consider having a comprehensive parasitology screening (described in Chapter 6.)

Natural remedies work effectively, as evidenced by re-testing, but you must stay on the therapy program outlined by a health-care practitioner for an initial 6-8 weeks and repeat as directed. I recommend preventive therapy of a parasite cleanse every year, and more often depending on risk factors.

I find the following non-drug therapy programs most effective:

1. Intestinal housecleaning (fiber bulking agents)

2. Natural substances for parasite removal

3. Intestinal "Rotor Rooter"

Intestinal Housecleaning

Especially in leaky gut, parasites have a perfect gastrointestinal environment in which to thrive: warm, damp, and dirty. The first step is to cleanse the gastrointestinal tract with a quality fiber-bulking agent. This is necessary to brush the lining of the intestinal wall and rid the body of parasites that are well established and attached. If this step is not taken, medications will not be effective because they cannot reach the worms until the encrusted waste matter and mucus protecting the worms are loosened or removed. This encrustation becomes a cozy protective housing for the parasites and must be removed to get to the core of the infestation.

The following natural ingredients are used in combinations to perform the scrubbing action: psyllium seed and husk, rice bran, alfalfa, citrus pectin, cascara sagrada, buckhorn bark, triphala, oat fiber, flax seed, bentonite clay, beet root, garlic, pumpkin seed, black walnut hulls, ficin. Many good fiber-bulking combinations are available. The product fulfilling this cleansing demand better than any I've used is Coloklysis™ Colon Cleanse from PhysioLogics®, described earlier. Once you begin the colon cleanse you will most likely pass thick strings of mucus, worms, and putrefied fecal matter. By removing these substances you are destroying the habitat that has been protecting these unwanted guests. See further details in "Colon Health—Waste Management" in this chapter.

Natural Substances for Parasite Removal

The following natural ingredients are extremely effective in removing parasites: Sweet Annie leaf and stem, garlic, Pau D'Arco bark and stem, black walnut hulls and husks, ficin, pumpkin seed, wormwood whole plant, plantain whole plant, gentian root, barberry root, Oregon grape root extract, and bromelain. It's been my experience that two herbal product combinations effectively eliminate parasitic infection: ParaCleanse® from PhysioLogics® and Parex™ Intensive Care from Metagenics®. Both formulas come in easy-to-swallow caplets and must be taken on an empty stomach.

Once an initial herbal therapy routine is completed, a homeopathic liquid complex is a beneficial follow-up course of therapy. A homeopathic is also useful for patients who cannot swallow pills, for small animals, children, and as an annual or semi-annual maintenance program. It is a liquid placed in water or juice and taken twice a day for a thirty-day course. The homeopathic herbal complex I prefer is formulated by DayStar Remedies, and available through health-care practitioners.

A combination product that includes ingredients to assist the bulking fiber agent in dealing with both parasites and Candida is Complete Cleanse™ by PhysioLogics®. It comes in a caplet form and is an effective addition to any fiber-bulking agent. What is unique to this product is that it contains a bi-layered caplet. The caplet has a three-stage release process: rapid release, secondary slow release, and extended release.

1. The rapid-release layer breaks down in the first part of the gastrointestinal tract. Here, an enzyme-activated herbal digestive blend helps start the process of healthy digestion and detoxification.

2. The second releases later in the lower part of the intestinal tract. This layer includes an enzyme-activated cleansing herb and fiber blend of butternut bark, beet fiber root, and flax seed. These are designed to promote the timely passage of partly digested food and waste through the lower part of the intestinal tract. Soothing herbs such as peppermint oil and licorice root are also added in the second layer. Also included in this layer are complexes composed of methyl-sulfonylmethane (MSM), garlic bulb, and black walnut leaf, which support the intestinal tract immune function.

3. The extended release layer includes a specially formulated probiotic flora replenishment complex that includes "friendly" bacteria and fructooligosaccharides (FOS).

With Complete Cleanse™, you don't have the inconvenience of mixing several ingredients for multiple detoxifying tasks. The recommended therapy, in conjunction with fiber bulking agents, is two caplets, twice a day.

Bentonite Clay is another substance effective in parasite removal. This substance is a clay-like volcanic ash used for centuries for its ability to absorb many times its weight in body toxins. It is my experience that a Bentonite-containing product should be introduced very slowly and in conjunction with a fiber-bulking product. If too much bentonite is introduced too early in the therapy, it can cause constipation and further backup and the subsequent circulation of toxic substances from a congested colon. One product easily available in health food stores that contains bentonite clay is Perfect Seven by Agape Health Products. Be sure to check with a health-care practitioner before introducing bentonite clay.

Intestinal "Rotor Rooter"

As previously mentioned, there are two effective ways to flush out old fecal matter, *Candida,* and parasites: colonic hydrotherapy and enemas. It is important to remember that as we loosen parasites, they must be fully eliminated. Colon hydrotherapy cleanses the entire length of the colon, all the way to the ileocecal valve, at the juncture of the small and large intestines. Enemas only reach the lower 12½ inches of the 5½-foot-long colon. Type of therapy will depend on the recommendation from a health-care practitioner, along with financial considerations and availability of qualified colon hydrotherapists in your area. (See "Resources" for a list of certified therapists worldwide.)

According to Great Smokies Diagnostic Laboratory, beneficial (friendly) bacteria should not be introduced into the intestinal system until after destroying any parasites and pathogens. Re-colonizing the bowel with friendly bacteria is a final step, taken only *after* the medications used have been clinically proven successful in eradicating the parasites.

A Word About Diet

According to most dietary experts, a diet high in simple carbohydrates like sugar, white flour, and processed foods provide the perfect environment for feeding parasites. These are not usually a consideration with leaky-gut patients, as they cannot tolerate them. We know that fiber-deficient foods may precipitate a breeding ground for parasites. These foods require more time to pass through the alimentary system. Slow transit time allows more food to decay and putrefy, thus producing stagnation in the colon that sets up the perfect living conditions for parasites and *Candida*. The challenge for victims of leaky gut is that our diets must contain the foods we can tolerate without allergic reactions, and consisting of natural sugars and carbohydrates from fruits, vegetables and tolerated grains. Therefore, I will refrain from giving

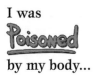
specific dietary recommendations regarding a parasitic cleansing diet, because it must be designed specifically for each individual by a qualified health-care professional.

A Note on Drug Therapies

Drug therapies can be effective; however, one must weigh the benefits against the adverse effects from the toxicity of such drugs. In the book, *Guess What Came to Dinner*, Ms. Gittleman provides a comprehensive list of anti-parasitic drugs and their side effects. The list includes physician references from *The Medical Letter on Drugs and Therapeutics*. Anyone wanting to expand his or her knowledge of parasitic infections would benefit from reading Ms. Gittleman's book.

Today, the traditional medical single-drug-course cure rate is less than 5 percent, and approximately half of the patients treated with drugs such as Flagyl (metronidazole) complain of side effects and refuse to take it again. Because of the low percentage of successful eradications with drugs, some physicians are now choosing to refer patients to natural therapies. These therapies are proven safer, gentler, and generally more effective.

Natural Relief from Nausea

Some patients experience slight nausea during the die-off of parasites. This symptom is generally experienced because of the toxic by-products released by the parasites into the body. There are several natural substances for relief.

Homeopathic dilution of ipecac syrup causes no adverse side effects and is successful in dealing with nausea. Concentrated ipecac syrup has been used for years to induce vomiting, but the homeopathic dilution has the reversed effect of calming. Be sure to check with a health-care practitioner for proper dosage and potency.

Aloe vera juice is another natural substance bringing immediate relief from nausea. Be sure to purchase a brand that must be refrigerated after opening and contains at least 70 percent pure aloe juice. Many brands use flavoring, such as apple or raspberry, to make it more appetizing; these ingredients are fine, if they don't include artificial coloring agents and the flavoring is natural.

Ginger extract, as mentioned earlier, is excellent for nausea. Place several drops in a glass of water and sip slowly. Fresh ginger tea is also effective, but does not bring relief as fast as extract diluted in water.

Depositing Reserves in Your pH Immune Account

Your saliva pH is a measurement of the alkaline/acid condition of your body. Maintaining an optimal pH level is essential for activating the digestive juices. The neutral pH is between 7.0 and 7.2. Keeping the body slightly alkaline discourages fungus, mold, *Candida* and parasites. All of these organisms thrive in an acid environment. Therefore, according to Dr. Bernard Jensen, the optimum pH for human tissue and blood plasma ranges from 7.35 to 7.45. As an example, distilled water is a pH of 7.0. Water pH can vary greatly depending on the source (I know of one valley in Washington State where the water is generally 8.5 pH, because of the basalt base rock). If the body is too acid or too alkaline, illness and disease can escalate. You can perform a pH test easily and economically at home by purchasing test strips available through a pharmacist. With leaky gut, it is best to test urine (not saliva) first thing in the morning and again at bedtime.

There's a lot of misconception about what is acid and what is alkaline. The acid-alkaline action is not necessarily related to how foods taste. For example, citrus fruits taste acidic and are alkaline-forming. Most protein foods such as meats, eggs, nuts, and dairy products are acid-forming. An interesting fact to digest is that while dairy products are acid-forming, whey from cow or goat's milk is alkaline-forming. The goat whey I've recommended for mineral/electrolyte replacement has the positive side effect of being alkaline-forming.

An alkaline ecosystem (in the intestinal flora) will create an unfriendly environment for uninvited organisms. Your diet should consist of 70 percent–80 percent alkaline-forming foods. It is also helpful to eat 50 percent of your daily food raw. This will allow for full benefits of enzymes, otherwise destroyed by cooking or heating.

At the onset of leaky gut, raw food other than in juices is not always tolerated, go slowly and pay attention to your symptoms. As your gut heals you'll be able to tolerate more and more raw foods.

➤ Flashback ➤

At first, I couldn't tolerate any raw foods. After three weeks of the primary elimination diet, I was able to add grated carrots and apples, if eaten slowly and in small quantities. Eventually I added any raw vegetable I could consume cooked.

The following is a basic guide to the acid- and alkaline-producing food groups:

Vegetables:

- All vegetables are alkaline-forming, including high-carbohydrate foods like potatoes, squash, and parsnips.

Grain:

- Most grains are acid-forming, except millet and buckwheat. Seeds and grains become more alkaline-forming if sprouted.

Vegetable and fruit juices:

- Most vegetable and fruit juices are highly alkaline-forming. Berry juices such as: huckleberry, raspberry, blackberry, elderberry, boysenberry, and currents are all alkaline-forming. However, strawberries and cranberries are acid-forming.

I was

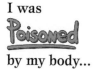

by my body...

172

Sugars:

- All sugars are acid forming with the exception of honey, which is alkaline-forming.

Meats, fish and dairy products

- All acid-forming.

8

Emotional Support

My intent in sharing this first-hand information is to assist you, and those who care about you, to regain a quality of life in a society that lives to eat, not eats to live. Is it easy? *No.* Is it possible? *Yes.*

Surviving in a Society That
Revolves Around Eating

One of the most challenging aspects of having food allergies is the potential social isolation as a result of the traditions revolved around eating. The history of gathering for a meal goes back two million years. Protohominid hunters and foragers divided food with their fellow hunters and their families. When we eat together, we bring our culture, customs, and expectations with us. It provides us the opportunity to converse and interact with others. For the person with leaky gut and food allergies, eating becomes not just a "food event," but also an event with complex challenges. However, the challenges lie in adjusting our attitudes and the attitudes of those with whom we socialize. Having to modify our eating surely does *not* have to keep people apart. On the contrary, it can be an opportunity to individualize and create new food events. It is a time to reflect and acknowledge our need to communicate with others, which is the true essence of gathering in the first place. It is a time for us to ask our social family for support in treating us as normal, not as people with a contagious disease. People with eating disorders are not contagious; they simply have specific requirements for the food they can safely consume. We are physically challenged, not emotionally impaired, even though at times we wonder if "our emotional cheese has slipped off its rice cracker!"

Allergies can be a divisive and isolating force in our society if we allow them to be. Be specific in asking for what you need from social situations. Express your desire to be included in gatherings, and that you'll bring your own food. Ask people close to you to refrain from attempts to convince you to "just have a little, it can't hurt." Explain that you understand they may feel awkward or even guilty consuming foods you can't. Assure them it's their companionship that's important to you, not what is consumed. Add some humor; tell them you're participating in a new food event called BYOF (bring your own food), it has a better sound than "pot luck", especially if the occasion is a bit more formal.

Be prepared to encounter individuals who have never been challenged with food allergies, who will say (or think) you're downright neurotic. They observe you eating foods they don't recognize and usually can't pronounce. To those individuals, I say, "I'm happy you have never experienced severe allergies, and I hope you never do." It's curious that eventually people start asking about the non-traditional, strange foods you're consuming. This provides a perfect opportunity to embark in new conversations, expanding their horizons and their vocabulary. Now you have an opportunity to bring something new to the dining table: conscious eating.

➤ Flashback ◆

The first Thanksgiving holiday after the onset of my illness was the most challenging. I invited twelve guests for a traditional, formal sit-down dinner. This event was particularly special because my youngest son was coming home to spend the holiday, for the first time in years. I was determined to fix a full dinner, even though I was unable to eat anything on the menu. I was still on a very limited diet, and I didn't want to risk a reaction from a newly introduced food. It was important to me to proceed with plans, regardless of my health challenges. It's not my style, or consciousness, to focus on my limitations, but it was difficult for me to cook the entire meal and not be able to taste.

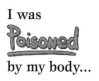
One of my guests, an art teacher, inquired beforehand as to what I could eat. "Organic carrots, rice, and apples," I responded.

When the time came to sit down to a full complement of food, she presented me with a work of art. She and her daughter had shredded organic carrots and sculptured an absolutely beautiful, detailed turkey. I was overwhelmed! The focus of the dinner was on my carrot turkey, not on my limitations, thanks to the thoughtfulness and sensitivity of special friends. I, too, had my holiday turkey, made from carrots. This was the true meaning of Thanksgiving, sharing and giving thanks, especially thanks for the kindness extended by caring friends.

Asking for What You Need: Help Others Help You

For some of us, asking for help is extremely difficult. Fortunately, I have a personal support system like none I've ever witnessed or encountered. Not everyone is as fortunate. The following components were, for me, the most important in structuring my support team: acknowledgement, privacy, and education.

Acknowledge the Fear

Fear as described by *Webster's* is "an unpleasant often strong emotion caused by anticipation or awareness of danger . . .. Fear is the most general term and implies anxiety and usually loss of courage (fear of the unknown)."

At the onset of any disease, fear is the first human response. LGS, MCSS/EI, and fibromyalgia are not acknowledged or understood by most conventional professionals, much less your personal support system. Be patient. Acknowledge your fear; it's the first step in coping with it. Express your concerns to your support team; it's the only way they can assist in diminishing some of your fears. It's amazing how some fears are monumental to us, yet to the support team they seem so basic, if they know what to deal with.

➤ Flashback ◄

My fears were, "Will I suffocate by not being able to swallow?" "What if I'm driving and I have a reaction?" "Where will I find the foods I can tolerate?" "I don't have enough energy to go shopping, much less locate specialty items." "Why don't my adult children understand this is life-threatening?"

My primary concern was finding a source of organic foods in the middle of winter in northern Idaho. I didn't have the energy to travel great distances in search of specialty sources. When I mentioned my dilemma to a friend, she immediately replied "I go into the city (125 miles away) every two weeks. I'd be happy to shop for whatever you need." And so, the personal shopper was created. Before long, I had friends and clients using her services as well. This single mother of three found a way to supplement her income. She trans-

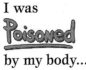
formed regular trips to a large city into a service for others who are challenged by poor health, lack of time, and/or adequate transportation.

Privacy

According to *Webster's*, privacy is "the quality or state of being apart from company or observation." Sometimes emotional support simply means giving you more space. This is especially evident when your body is experiencing so many physical changes and requiring special considerations on a daily basis. It's not like you drink juice in the morning, take your supplements, and you're okay for the rest of the day. You are forced to embark on a 24-hour-a-day challenge, a complete life-style change.

Explain to the people you care about, and those that care about you, that sometimes you just need to have personal quiet time to reflect, heal, and take stock of your situation. It is *not* helpful for someone like a well-meaning neighbor, friend, or relative to chat, visit, or ask for daily reports on your condition. This is energy we just don't have to give. I assess the situation by asking, "Is this experience going to be a taker or giver of energy?" If the situation is too *energy-consuming* then I gracefully bow out or become unavailable. There may be situations when you need to express that the best help comes in the form of simply giving you space.

➤ Flashback ◄

The first few months were so challenging for me, I had to detach from well-meaning friends. I was in

*colon hydrotherapy. I self-administered enemas. I
maintained my consulting practice. I continued
medical writing and research. I had therapeutic
massage and lymphatic stimulation weekly. I
juiced daily, and experimented with every food
and food preparation method I could get my hands
on. Living became overwhelming, a full-time job,
and with only a quarter of my usual energy.*

People outside your household who can't, or
don't choose to, contribute by assisting in daily
necessary tasks (shopping for organic foods, pre-
paring the food for juicing, juicing, cooking, etc.)
should be emotionally supportive by respecting
your need for space. If you agree to anything less,
you'll pay the huge price of adding toxic emotions
of disappointment and anxiety to your already
toxic body.

Education

Educating is to "provide with information"
(Webster's). Ask those who care about you to read
all they can regarding digestive disorders, food allergies, *Candida*, parasites, drug side-effects and
multiple chemical sensitivities. Give them a copy of
this book. Explain the choices you've made in taking control of your health-care. Allow them
permission to disagree with your decision, but
communicate your desire for them to respect your
choice. If they choose to continue pursuing their
point of view, don't feed their negativity. Usually,
the people quickest to express an opinion are the

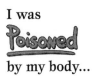
ones least informed. *To the uninformed, anything less than drug therapy must be "quackery."* It soon becomes evident these people know nothing of the alternative natural-healing modalities used and written about for centuries. They are accustomed to quick fixes. Wholistic medicine is not quick. However, it *is* effective and the investment pays higher dividends than symptom-care. Remember, you are not asking permission, you are expressing a decision. If they choose not to be supportive, respect their position, fade out of their life, and find a new support team.

Many individuals, clients and non-clients, contacted me when they heard I was writing about leaky gut, fibromyalgia, and the resulting multiple chemical sensitivities. I was constantly asked to write about guidance in dealing with people who are not informed about natural health and have no idea about the seriousness of these conditions. Their suggestions, blended with my experiences, helped to formulate this chapter. I am honored they chose to share their stories of personal challenge.

9

Living with the Effects of Leaky Gut

Reaction-Emergency Preparedness

Each person has individual responses and needs. *Do not* attempt to control allergic reactions without the assistance and ongoing support of your physician and health-care practitioner.

An acute attack can begin suddenly, peaking within minutes, or develop gradually over hours or days. Death can occur because patients, or those around them, do not realize the severity of the reaction. Prolonged stressful respiratory restriction is difficult for the functioning of the entire body. You must begin to manage the attack at the *earliest sign* of reaction.

- Have a plan worked out with your physician, health-care practitioner, and those close to you on how to handle an emergency.
- Be sure to have a medical consent and keep it updated.
- Give copies of your medical consent to everyone authorized to make decisions on your behalf.
- Alert family members, co-workers, close friends, and neighbors about your condition.

- Be specific regarding your needs, what action to take, and who to contact if a reaction occurs.
- If someone does not take your condition seriously, don't try to convince them, ask someone else.
- Keep a copy of your medical information and medical consent in your car or briefcase and wear a medical alert bracelet or necklace; it may save your life.

How I "Get Out" of an
Allergic Reaction

I use the following steps to "get out" of my reactions to food or environmental causes, Naturally:

1. I remove myself from the suspected food or pollutant immediately. If ingested: I discontinue eating the food or substance. If environmental: I get out immediately into clean, fresh air.

2. I use a homeopathic remedy formulated specifically for allergic reactions by DayStar Remedies (see product reference). I administer six drops directly under the tongue and repeat every five to eight minutes, as needed. The emergency reaction subsides within eight to twelve minutes.

3. I *always* carry an emergency kit to be as prepared as possible. Besides my homeopathic remedy, my kit contains emergency injectable

epinephrine (Adrenaline) and an inhaler, prescribed by my medical doctor. I have *never* had to use the epinephrine, as the homeopathic remedy has been very successful in controlling my reactions. I did use the inhaler at the onset of my leaky gut, until an effective natural remedy could be identified. My kit also contains a charcoal mask, in the event I get into a situation that is not safe environmentally.

4. I alert someone around me that I'm having a reaction. This is extremely important because if the reaction escalates and I can't speak for myself, someone must be available to call for help.

5. If the reaction is from an environmental source, I shower and wash my hair at the first possible opportunity. This is critical to minimize absorption of the offending substance and reduce toxic overload.

6. After an acute reaction, it is important to cleanse the gastrointestinal tract. I schedule a session for colon hydrotherapy as soon as possible. I'm fortunate that there are now two colon therapists within my vicinity. There were times when I had to call the therapist and exclaim, "I'm having an acute reaction, I'm on my way." As soon as colon therapy was administered, my reactions disappeared. If I'm not able to have colon hydrotherapy, I administer enemas. Enemas provide some reaction relief, but there's no comparison to the immediate relief of colon hydrotherapy.

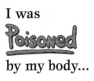
7. After a reaction, from food or environmental exposure, I maintain a liquid diet for 1–2 days. The diet consists of fresh juices, rice protein drinks, herbal teas, and supplementation with mineral whey. This regime allows the body systems to use the energy for detoxifying and gives the digestive system a rest.

8. I take additional buffered Vitamin C because of its ability to reduce an allergic reaction. It assists in boosting the immune system by producing lymphocytes. Vitamin C prevents free-radical damage and is used by the thymus gland (involved in immunity) to increase the mobility of phagocyte cells, which "eat" bacteria, viral cells, and other harmful foreign substances. After a reaction, I take a dose of 2000–3000 mg of Vitamin C. Normally I take 4000 mg as a total daily dose. I continue higher levels of Vitamin C intake for 3–4 days after the reaction. For the leaky gut patient, it is important to find individual tolerance levels and to *always* take Vitamin C with food. Taking it on an empty stomach may cause stomach or G.I. discomfort. A health-care practitioner can assist in finding your individual tolerance level and the right complex.

9. I increase my consumption of a complete Vitamin B complex with folic acid. I take a daily total of 500 mg of B complex (which includes 400 mcg of folic acid per 100 mg.). I continue this for two days, then return to my mainte-

nance dose of one 100 mg tablet three times daily, with meals. Vitamin B plays an important role in the health of the gastrointestinal tract and nervous system, is needed for healthy blood, and produces red blood cells and antibodies. Folic acid assists the immune system by increasing the ability to recognize invading microbes and strengthening white blood cells. If the reaction is acute accompanied by extreme fatigue, I also use a Vitamin B-12 Liposome sublingual spray manufactured by PhysioLogics.

10. I take a homeopathic complex, formulated by DayStar Remedies, to provide liver support. This complex reduces the accompanying liver pain of toxic overload. I take 6 drops under the tongue 4–6 times daily after a reaction. Once the liver pain subsides, I use this formula for maintenance support by taking 6 drops every evening (see product reference).

11. I use an air purifier with a four-stage filtration system (pre-filter, HEPA, activated carbon, Zeolite) in my home, office, and car.

12. I stay in my "safe" areas (home and office) for 1–2 days, until all lingering effects of the reaction have disappeared. This is imperative because the body needs time to detoxify and repair.

13. Most of all, I do whatever I can to reduce stress and stressful situations. Stress, combined with a reaction, compromises the already overworked immune system by adding to your total accumulated exposure (TAE).

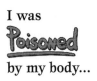
14. I lower my expectations and allow my body time to recuperate. At first, it was difficult to grant myself permission to slow down. My mind was operating at the usual fast pace, but my body couldn't keep up. This situation encouraged me to create the phrase, "My mind is writing checks my body can't cash."

Note: I also have a portable oxygen tank in my office and home. This is critical if an environmental exposure occurs and emergency measures are needed. It is also important for clearing acute "brain-fog." Check with your health-care provider for guidance in acquiring a tank and using it properly.

My Battered Ration Crate

Travel is, for most of us, inevitable. Travel has a significant meaning in each person's life-style. For the purposes of this book, I'll deal with every-day travel as required to and from our place of employment and everyday necessities. Traveling abroad or for long distances would require careful advance planning, and special accommodations (see "Business and Overnight Trips" in this chapter).

My business partner creatively assembled a plastic crate, with a tight fitting cover, for my on-the-go food. Some of the items I found invaluable include:

- Brown rice cakes
- Brown rice crackers
- Almonds (as tolerated)
- Supplemental protein powder

- Spoon, fork, small spreading knife, small sharp knife
- Glass canning jar and lid (to use as shaker for protein drink)
- Small bowl and plate (wood or ceramic)
- Small pill container with digestive enzymes
- Small containers of organic applesauce
- Small single-serving containers of rice or almond milk (this doesn't need to be refrigerated until opened)
- Individual serving cans of organic juices (as tolerated)
- Plenty of napkins
- Small bags to use for garbage
- Bottles of pure drinking water
- Disposable hand wipes (natural, unscented) or a washcloth in a plastic bag

In California we called kits like these "earthquake survival kits," in Idaho they're called "snow survival kits." Same purpose: taking care of your needs when other resources are not readily available. Even if you don't live in an area as rural as I do, it's not always convenient to locate a store with an organic food department at the time you need it. For those of us with food and/or chemical sensitivities, the challenge is not only finding the foods we can tolerate, they must be organic (there is a profound difference). Being prepared is essential, it *puts us back in control,* and that's important at a time when everything in our health and environment is so out of control.

➤ Flashback ➤

I've experienced panic at being away from my food sources and not able to get home soon enough to keep my body from experiencing a negative reaction. I remember having to make a trip to a major city some 125 miles away. I thought I packed enough food for the day. All the appointments took much longer than anticipated, and by early evening I was out of food. *The health-food stores were closed and restaurants weren't an option. I finally resorted to buying some rice milk and rice cakes from an all-night grocery store. No, it wasn't a meal, but it got me through the emergency. That incident was what encouraged my business partner to assemble the "on-the-go" crate for me. Never again was I caught without the most basic needs.*

My Battered Ice Chest

It's a good thing I drive a sport utility vehicle, because I need room for my attachès. An ice chest is another necessity for traveling away from home. Since you'll probably be cooking extra quantities of food for your trip, whether for a few hours or several days, it's important to store it properly. All too often we hear of food poisoning from improper refrigeration and the resulting bacteria.

I have a client who had dinner at a restaurant on a hot August day, and took home the leftovers (without an ice chest). The trip home was thirty minutes and the car was air-conditioned. She immediately refrigerated the leftover food upon arrival home. The next evening she decided to eat the leftovers. Later that night the effects of food poisoning hit: acute stomach pain, vomiting, and diarrhea. Next came the necessary trip to the emergency room and I.V. therapy. That dinner cost her over $1,200 and a potentially life-threatening situation. Isn't an ice chest worth the small investment of $20 to $100? A leaky-gut patient already has a weakened immune system. Add to it food poisoning, and this could truly be your most expensive meal and perhaps your *last supper.* Whatever foods you are currently tolerating, cook extra quantities and carry some with you. When away from my local area, I carry rice milk for my protein drinks, leftovers, fresh vegetables, and juices.

Business and Overnight Trips

I have many LGS clients who travel extensively for business. They resort to carrying a soft-sided insulated chest as part of their allowed carry-on baggage. The prepared foods are previously frozen and act as the cooling agent. Planning ahead allows them to fit into a normal life-style.

When obtaining lodging, be sure to ask if they have facilities to warm and refrigerate food. If the facility has a restaurant, ask to speak with the food-service manager or chef. Explain your special dietary needs. Many facilities will accommodate your re-

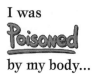
quests. Also inquire if they would cook for you if you provide the food. It's amazing what you get if you ask for it! Don't be embarrassed, millions of people have special dietary and environmental needs, and establishments are more and more willing to cooperate with individualized needs. Carrying or purchasing your own food allows you to travel with confidence; you know the ingredients of everything you consume.

The following suggestions for traveling are my personal preferences and those submitted by clients:

- Frozen organic vegetables: peas, green beans, spinach, chard, corn, bean sprouts, celery, chopped onions and garlic. I chop and freeze small bags of onions and minced or juiced frozen garlic, to add to stir fries and omelets. Be sure to freeze in small quantities or for a single meal.

- Frozen cooked grains: brown rice, brown basmati rice, quinoa.

  Don't overcook for freezing, leave a little al dente. When reheated it can be stir fried or steamed. Place just enough grain in a bag for a single serving.

- Frozen spinach or veggie patties.

  I make up some chard patties (sautéed onions, chard, garlic, rice, bread crumbs, egg, 1 drop of *Stevia,* and herbs) and pan-fry. They are a great hot main course or tasty eaten cold. I've served them to guests and they can't believe they're eating a meatless patty.

Get creative. Turn your necessity into a new gourmet experience. You may be pleasantly surprised by the curiosity expressed and the interesting conversations that result, naturally.

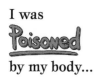
Afterword

Modern conventional medicine performs miracles and saves lives, especially in the case of injury or trauma. I am a prime example; clot-dissolving drugs saved my life after a traumatic injury. Doctors perform daily miracles by repairing physical damage and removing (and often replacing) diseased organs. However, conventional medicine has little to offer an individual with digestive diseases, environmental illness, and chronic disorders. Physicians are trained to turn off a reaction with drugs for symptom-care, but in the process, can perpetuate a self-destructive cycle masking the root causes.

The new breed of health-care practitioners and medical doctors employ methods advocated by Hippocrates. They emphasize diet, nutrients, non-toxic treatments, environmental modifications, and therapies that encourage the healing process, and reserve drugs and surgery as a last resort. I salute these health-care professionals who work tirelessly to seek the causes of disease and advocate true health-care, naturally.

What's Next?

Dr. Gilbère is completing her next book titled "MCS: First-Hand Solutions to Second-Hand Reactions"—the book starts where this leaves off. It provides a handy "urgent care guide" for dealing with allergic reactions of all kinds. It's arranged by situations, symptoms and solutions—covering everything you need to know to help yourself, or a loved one, through the fear, panic, pain and danger of an allergic reaction, naturally.

She has completed her book "Invisible Illnesses", now available. It uncovers the progressive development of, and solutions for, "medically unexplainable", chronic conditions.

Dr. Gilbère writes weekly newspaper articles titled "Second Hand Reactions" published and circulated throughout the U.S., Canada and Europe. Her articles are for the purpose of education and to provide support to the millions afflicted with allergies and multiple chemical sensitivities. If you'd like to view her articles you may do so on her website at: www.drgloriagilbere.com.

Please DO NOT email for advice. If you choose to consult with her, you may contact her office at (208) 255-1920. The office will make the appropriate arrangements for a telephone consultation or an appointment at the health center in Sandpoint, Idaho. Her office is located 78 miles northeast of Spokane, WA, 45 miles north of Coeur d'Alene, ID and 70 miles south of the Canadian border (Creston, B.C.).

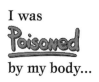
Resources for Testing

Great Smokies Diagnostic Laboratories

18A Regent Park Blvd.
Asheville, NC 28806
Tel: (800) 522-4762

Provides the following assessments: Gastrointestinal, Immunology, Nutritional, Endocrinology, Metabolic.

Diagnos-Techs, Inc.

6620 S. 192nd Place, Bldg. J
Kent, WA 98032
Tel: (800) 878-3787

Provides the following analyses: Yeast Screens, Digestion Efficiency Panel, GI Pathogen Tests, Melatonin BioRhythm and Challenge Test, NTx Bone Marker Test, Mucosal Barrier Screens, Adrenal Stress Markers, Hormone Panels, Gastro-Intestinal Health Panel.

Doctor's Data

P.O. Box 111
West Chicago, IL 608186-0111
Tel: (800) 323-2784

Provides the following: Hair Elements Analysis, Whole Blood Elements Analysis, Packed Red Blood Cell Elements Analysis, Urine Elements Analysis, Creatinine Clearance, Urine D-Glucaric and Mercapturic Acid Analyses, Urine and Plasma Amino Acids Analyses, Fecal Toxic Elements, Intestinal Barrier Function Test.

Meridian Valley Clinical Laboratory
24030 132nd Ave SE
Kent, WA 98042
Tel: (800) 234-6825

Provides the following analyses: DHEA Screening Blood Lectin Serotypes, Elisa Allergy Tests, Blood Mineral Analysis, Urine Mineral Analysis, Hair Mineral Analysis, Comprehensive Digestive Stool Analysis, Essential Amino Acid Testing, Adrenal Steroids, Parasitology, Essential Fatty Acids, Fractionated Estrogens.

Immuno Laboratories Inc.
1620 W. Oakland Park Blvd.
Ft. Lauderdale, FL 33311
Tel: (800) 231-9197

Provides the following analyses: IgE Airborne & Food Allergy Assay, Candida Albicans Assay, Epstein Barr Virus Profile, Helicobacter Pylori Assay, and Essential Metabolics Analysis through SpectraCell Labs.

Serammune Physicians Laboratory
1890 Preston White Drive, 2nd floor
Reston, VA 22091
Tel: (800) 553-5472

Provides Comprehensive Food and Environmental Blood Testing through the Elisa/Act Test. The Elisa/Act Test measures over 300 foods, environmental chemicals, preservatives, mercury sensitivity, and three major classes of yeasts.

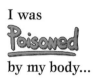
Ordering Referenced Products:

For your convenience, the professional products recommended may be ordered by credit card or pre-paid directly from DoctorsChoice, Naturally toll free at: 1-866-698-1581. This service is provided solely for the purpose of ordering products referred to in this book.

New Clients:

To consult with Dr. Gilbere either by telephone or at her health center in northern Idaho, you must call 208-255-1920 (PST), or fax a request for new client information to 208-265-8805.

Resources

International Association for Colon Hydrotherapy (I-ACT), P.O. Box 461285, San Antonio, TX 78246-1285 USA, (210) 366-2888, e-mail: iact@healthy.net, www.i-act.org, Association for Certification of Colon Hydrotherapists.

Nutritional Ecological & Environmental Delivery Systems (NEEDS), P.O. Box 580, E. Syracuse, NY 13057 USA, (800) 634-1380, www.needs.com, Vitamins, supplements, air/water purification systems, domestics, books.

Bibliography

Several hundred books, articles, world-wide-web sites and manuscripts were reviewed and studied in the writing of this book. The following is only a representative sampling of these resources.

Balch, Dr. James F. and Phyllis A. Balch, C.N.C. *Prescription for Nutritional Healing.* Garden City Park, NY: Avery Publishing Group, 1994

BBC News. *Bowel Cancer: The silent killer.* England: Online Network, 1998

Bland, Dr. Jeffrey. *Medical Applications of Clinical Nutrition.* New Canaan, CT: Keats Publishing, 1983

Bland, Dr. Jeffrey. *The Inflammatory Disorders.* Washington: Health Comm Seminar Series, 1997

Buchman, Dian Dincin. *Herbal Medicine.* New York, NY: Gramercy Publishing Co., 1980

Canary Connect News. Coralville, IA: Canary Connect Publications, 1998

Carter, Mildred. *Body Reflexology.* West Nyack, NY: Parker Publishing Co., 1983

Cichoke, Dr. Anthony. *The Complete Book of Enzyme Therapy.* Garden City Park, NY: Avery Publishing Group, 1999

Crook, Dr. William. *The Yeast Connection.* New York, NY: Vintage Books, 1986

The Drug and Natural Medicine Advisor. Richmond, VA: Time Life Custom Publishing, 1997

Dumke, Nicolette. *Allergy Cooking with Ease.* Lancaster, PA: Starburst Publishers, 1992

Dumke, Nicolette. *5 Years without Food, The Food Allergy Survival Guide.* Louisville, CO: Adapt Books, 1997

Ewing, W.N. and D.J.A. Cole. *The Living Gut.* England: Redwood Books, 1994

Gittleman, Ann Louise. *Guess What Came to Dinner-Parasites and Your Health.* Garden City Park, NY: Avery Publishing Group, 1993

Golan, Dr. Ralph. *Optimal Wellness.* New York, NY: Ballantine Books, 1995

Golos, Natalie, and Golos Frances Golbitz. *If This is Tuesday, It Must be Chicken.* New Canaan, CT: Keats Publishing, 1983

Gray, Robert. *The Colon Health Handbook.* Reno, NV: Emerald Publishing, 1991

Haas, Dr. Elson. *Staying Healthy with the Seasons.* Berkeley, CA: Celestial Arts, 1981

Heimlich, Jane. *What Your Doctor Won't Tell You.* New York, NY: Harper Perennial, 1990

Heinerman, John. *Heinerman's Encyclopedia of Healing Juices.* West Nyack, NY: Parker Publishing Company, 1994

Jamison, Dr. Alcinous. *Intestinal Ills.* New York, NY: Chas. Tyrrell M.D., 1917

Jensen, Dr. Bernard. *Tissue Cleansing Through Bowel Managment.* Escondido, CA: Bernard Jensen Enterprises, 1981.

Kellogg, Dr. John Harvey. *Colon Hygiene.* Battle Creek, MI: Modern Medicine Publishing Co., 1923

Kenton, L., and S. Kenton. *Raw Energy.* London: Century Publishing, 1984

Ley, Beth. *Castor Oil: Its Healing Properties.* Aliso Viejo, CA: BL Publications, 1989

Lipski, Elizabeth. *Digestive Wellness.* New Canaan, CT: Keats Publishing, 1996

Loes, Dr. Michael, and David Steinman, M.A. *The Aspirin Alternative*. Topanga, CA: Freedom Press, 1999

Loomis, Dr. Howard. *Enzymes, The Key to Health*. Madison, WI: 21st Century Nutrition Publication, 1999

Lopez, Dr. D.A., Dr. R.M. Williams, and Dr. K. Miehlke. *Enzymes: The Fountain of Life*. Charleston, SC: The Neville Press, 1994

Losenvold, Dr. Lloyd. *Can a Gluten-Free Diet Help?* New Canaan, CT: Keats Publishing, 1992

Lust, John. *Drink Your Troubles Away*. New York, NY: Benedict Lust Publications, 1967

The Merck Manual of Medical Information. Whitehouse Station, N.J.: Merck Research Laboratories, 1997

McWilliams, Peter, and John Roger. *You Can't Afford the Luxury of a Negative Thought*. Los Angeles, CA: Prelude Press, 1988

Millard, Dr. F.P., and Dr. A.G. Walmsley. *Applied Anatomy of the Lymphatics*. Mokelumne Hill, CA: Health Research, 1964

MFA Collection. Coeur d'Alene, ID: MAST Enterprises, 1986

MuCos. Oral Enzymes. Germany: Mucos Pharma Gmbh & Co., 1992

Physicians' Desk Reference, 50th Edition: Medical Economics Company, 1996

Rogers, Dr. Sherry. *You Are What You Ate*. Syracuse, NY: Prestige Publishing, 1997

Rogers, Dr. Sherry. *The E.I. Syndrome*. Syracuse, NY: Prestige Publishers, 1986

Rogers, Dr. Sherry. *Wellness against All Odds*. Syracuse, NY: Prestige Publishing, 1994

Schmidt, Michael A., Lendon H. Smith, and Keith W. Sehnert. *Beyond Antibiotcs, 50 (or so) Ways to Boost Immunity and Avoid Antibiotics*. Berkeley, CA: North Atlantic Books, 1993

Shabert, Dr. Judy, and Nancy Ehrlich. *The Ultimate Nutrient Glutamine*. Garden City Park, NY: Avery Publishing Group, 1994

Special Report: Aloe Vera & You. Orlando, FL: Pinnacle Printing, 1994

Stoll, Dr. Walt. *Saving Yourself from the Disease-Care Crisis*. Panama City, FL: Sunrise Health Coach, 1996

Tenney, Louise, M.H. *Colon Health*. Pleasant Grove, UT: Woodland Publishing, 1998

Thie, John. *Touch for Health*. Marina del Ray, CA: DeVorss and Company, 1995

Truss, Dr. Orian. *The Missing Diagnosis*. Birmingham, AL: The Missing Diagnosis, Inc., 1983

United States Pharmacopeia, The. Rockville, MD: United States Pharmacopeial Convention, 1995

Van der Hulst, RRWJ. *Glutamine, an essential nutrient for the gut*. University of Maastricht, Germany: 1996

Walker, Dr. Norman. *Colon Health*. Prescott, AZ: Norwalk Press, 1995

Weinberger, Stanley, C.M.T. *Parasites—An Epidemic in Disguise*. Larkspur, CA: Healing Within, 1993

Weiss, Jennifer, N.D., and Burnett Vena N.D. *Colon Cleansing, The Best-Kept Secret*. Auburn, CA: The Sunshine Company, 1989

Wigmore, Ann. *The Wheatgrass Book*. Garden City Park, NY: Avery Publishing Group, 1985

Index

Index

Index

About the Author

Dr. Gilbère is a natural health practitioner, ergonomist, medical writer, and researcher. She maintains a private practice in northern Idaho and is Director of the Naturopathic Health and Research Center. Her services include clinical work, telephone consultations (nationally and internationally) with clients and physicians, teaching, and lecturing. Dr. Gilbère writes numerous articles for 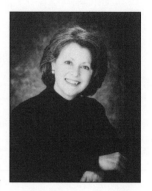 newspapers, health magazines, and trade journals, including a regular column, "Second Hand Reactions," published in the U.S. and Canada.

Dr. Gilbère is a keynote presenter and has conducted seminars on varied disciplines of wholistic health in the U.S., Canada, China, Argentina, Spain, and England.

As a consultant, educator, and trainer in preventive health-care, environmental color psychology, and EcoErgonomics, her client list includes Fortune 500 companies, universities, hospitals, health-care organizations, government agencies, school districts, corporations, small businesses, and professional associations.

She is internationally respected as a natural-medicine researcher, environmental health consultant, writer, and an authoritative influence in the discovery of the causes, effects, and natural solutions for leaky gut syndromes and chemically induced immune system disorders.

For information regarding her consulting services, speaking engagements, or interviews call (208) 255-1920 (Mon.-Thurs. 9:00 to 4:00 Pacific Time).

E-mail: info@drgloriagilbere.com, visit her web site at: www.drgloriagilbere.com. She can be contacted by writing:

Dr. Gloria Gilbère
316 N. 2nd Ave. Courtyard
Suite "D"
Sandpoint, Idaho 83864 USA